D0742085

November 17, 2015

The Soul of Medicine

To Mason,

Welcome my "little brother" to the Boston Medical Community for Jesus Christ. You're now the newest member of my Christian Medical Family. Like the Hotel California, you can check out anytime you like, but you can never leave." May this book bless you and others, the way it has blessed me.

Love & Blessings,

John

The Soul of Medicine

Spiritual Perspectives and Clinical Practice

EDITED BY

John R. Peteet, M.D.

AND

Michael N. D'Ambra, M.D.

Harvard Medical School
Boston, Massachusetts

The Johns Hopkins University Press
BALTIMORE

 Published 2011
Printed in the United States of America on acid-free paper
9 8 7 6 5 4 3 2 1

The Johns Hopkins University Press
2715 North Charles Street
Baltimore, Maryland 21218-4363
www.press.jhu.edu

Library of Congress Cataloging-in-Publication Data
The soul of medicine : spiritual perspectives and clinical practice / edited by John R. Peteet and Michael N. D'Ambra.
p. ; cm.
Includes bibliographical references and index.
ISBN-13: 978-1-4214-0299-4 (hardcover : alk. paper)
ISBN-10: 1-4214-0299-8 (hardcover : alk. paper)
1. Medicine. 2. Medicine—Religious aspects. 3. Mind and body. I. Peteet, John R., 1947– II. D'Ambra, Michael N.
[DNLM: 1. Spirituality. 2. Religion and Medicine. WM 61]
R708.S68 2011
201′.661—dc22 2011009990

A catalog record for this book is available from the British Library.

Special discounts are available for bulk purchases of this book. For more information, please contact Special Sales at 410-516-6936 or specialsales@press.jhu.edu.

The Johns Hopkins University Press uses environmentally friendly book materials, including recycled text paper that is composed of at least 30 percent post-consumer waste, whenever possible.

Contents

Contributors

Gowri Anandarajah, M.D., Professor (Clinical), Department of Family Medicine, Brown University School of Medicine, Providence, Rhode Island; gowri_anandarajah@mhri.org

Michael J. Balboni, M.Div., Th.M., Ph.D., Center for Psycho-oncology and Palliative Care Research, Dana-Farber Cancer Institute, Boston, Massachusetts; mjbalboni@partners.org

Tracy A. Balboni, M.D., M.P.H., Assistant Professor of Radiation Oncology, Harvard Medical School, Boston, Massachusetts; tbalboni@partners.org

Terry R. Bard, D.D., Clinical Instructor of Psychiatry, Harvard Medical School, Beth Israel Deaconess Medical Center, Boston, Massachusetts; Terry_Bard@hms.harvard.edu

Michael N. D'Ambra, M.D., Associate Professor of Anesthesiology, Harvard Medical School, Brigham and Women's Hospital, Boston, Massachusetts; mdambra@partners.org

Christine J. Driessen, C.S.B., M.A., M.S.T., J.D., Christian Science Practitioner, Church of Christ, Scientist, New York, New York; driessencsb@gmail.com

Areej El-Jawahri, M.D., Clinical Fellow in Medicine, Harvard Medical School, Boston, Massachusetts; ael-jawahri@partners.org

Marta D. Herschkopf, M.St., M.D., Resident Physician (Psychiatry), New York University School of Medicine, New York, New York; marta.herschkopf@nyumc.org

Travis D. Johnson, M.D., M.P.H., Faculty, Hendersonville Family Medicine Residency Program, University of North Carolina, Hendersonville, North Carolina; travisduanejohnson@gmail.com

Walter Kim, Ph.D., Associate Minister/Teaching Pastor, Park Street Church, Boston, Massachusetts; wkim@parkstreet.org

John R. Knight, M.D., Associate Professor of Pediatrics, Harvard Medical School, Senior Associate in Medicine/Associate in Psychiatry, Children's Hospital, Boston, Massachusetts; john.knight@childrens.harvard.edu

Shan W. Liu, M.D., S.D., Instructor in Surgery, Harvard Medical School, Department of Emergency Medicine, Massachusetts General Hospital, Boston, Massachusetts; sliu1@partners.org

Walter Moczynski, D.Min., M.T.S., M.Div., Instructor in Ministry, Harvard Divinity School, Dana-Farber Cancer Institute, Boston, Massachusetts; wmoczynski@partners.org

John R. Peteet, M.D., Associate Professor of Psychiatry, Harvard Medical School, Brigham and Women's Hospital, Boston, Massachusetts; jpeteet @partners.org

David C. Ring, M.D., Ph.D., Associate Professor of Orthopedic Surgery, Harvard Medical School, Boston, Massachusetts; dring@partners.org

Steven C. Schachter, M.D., Professor of Neurology, Harvard Medical School, Director of Research, Department of Neurology, Beth Israel Deaconess Medical Center, Boston, Massachusetts; sschacht@bidmc.harvard.edu

Jon Schiller, M.D., Valley Medical Group, Amherst, Massachusetts; joschill04 @gmail.com

Elizabeth Spencer-Smith, M.D., F.A.C.R., Rheumatology Associates, Greenbrae, California; foxydoxy9@yahoo.com

Robert Wall, M.Div., M.S.N., F.N.P.-B.C., A.P.M.H.N.P.-B.C., Commonwealth Care Alliance, Boston, Massachusetts; wall.r@comcast.net

Preface

Biomedicine continues to contribute importantly to the treatment of disease, but there is widespread concern that medicine may be losing its soul. As technology, commercialization, and government and insurer bureaucracies impinge on the doctor-patient relationship, both patient satisfaction and physician morale have declined. At the same time interest has grown in the spiritual dimension of medicine and health.

Americans spend about $1.5 billion annually on books on spirituality and religion, and about 40 percent have sought out complementary and alternative therapies. Medline contains 5,000 citations on spirituality in relation to health research. Recognizing the relevance of spirituality to patient care, national regulatory agencies and policy organizations such as the Joint Commission have mandated attention to patient spirituality as part of routine clinical care. Screening patients using survey instruments such as the FICA Spiritual History Tool (*f*aith and belief, the *i*mportance of faith, the *c*ommunity of faith, and *a*ddressing faith in care) is becoming increasingly common. In 2004, 84 U.S. medical schools offered courses in spirituality and medicine.* Yet there is a lack of consensus about the clinical implications of this spirituality movement. What if any spiritual information should be part of a physician's standard assessment of a patient? How should a physician respond to a patient who refuses life-saving care on religious grounds? Should a physician pray with a patient? Such questions raise deeper ones about the goals of medicine, the nature of healing, and the physician's role in responding to patients who experience reality through different worldviews.

One major obstacle to working and teaching in this area has been the lack of a shared understanding of spirituality. Individuals often approach spirituality as the proverbial blind men explored the elephant, each using a favored

* A. H. Fortin and K. G. Barnett, "Medical school curricula in spirituality and medicine," *JAMA* 291 (2004): 2883.

paradigm. A religious believer might approach spirituality as a window into a supernatural realm; an atheist as a psychological phenomenon, understandable in naturalistic terms; a sociologist as an aspect of cultural diversity; a psychologist as a means of coping; an existentialist as a way of finding meaning; and an open-minded agnostic as mystery. Lack of consensus complicates discussions of the relationship between spirituality and health.

We suggest that whereas the term *religion* generally denotes a tradition of beliefs and practices shared by a community, *spirituality* is a more inclusive term that refers to a person's connection with a larger or transcendent reality that gives life meaning. This could range from awe in the face of nature to hope for immortality through scientific discovery. A person can be spiritual without being religious or be religious without being spiritual. But even individuals who do not consider themselves spiritual or religious have a philosophy of life or a "worldview," which Freud defined as "an intellectual construction which solves all the problems of our existence uniformly on the basis of one overriding hypothesis."*

As co-directors of the Harvard Medical School course "Spirituality and Healing in Medicine," we became aware of the need for a basic text to prepare students for dealing with the spiritual, worldview, and related moral dimensions of the interaction between physician and patient. Ideally, such a text would help students address the ways in which their own worldviews relate to professionalism and help provide a fulcrum for making the pivotal transition from student to physician. We hope that this book fills such needs by focusing attention on the clinical relevance of patients' and clinicians' spirituality. We have included both religious and secular perspectives, and illustrative case examples to supplement conceptual discussions.

The chapters parallel the organization of the course we have been teaching for a number of years. Part I sets these issues within a historical and clinical context. In Chapter 1, Michael Balboni and Tracy Balboni review the historical relationship between spirituality and medicine, highlighting current challenges. In Chapter 2, writing as a psychiatrist, an anesthesiologist, and a theologian, we suggest a framework for approaching spirituality in a range of clinical contexts.

Part II presents the relationships of the major traditions to modern medi-

*S. Freud, "The question of a Weltanshauung," in *New Introductory Lectures on Psychoanalysis* (New York: Norton, 1933), p. 1.

cine. Chapters 3 through 11 address the following questions from the perspective of the authors' worldviews:

1. What narrative or idea in your tradition helps to define the ultimate nature and essential concerns of human beings?
2. What resources for living well does your tradition offer? What insights about life and healing does your tradition provide?
3. How does your tradition challenge or reinforce contemporary medical practice?
4. How do faith and culture influence each other in your tradition?
5. How do you access and address spirituality in your clinical practice? How do your beliefs influence your practice?

We chose some traditions and not others based on those that we and our North American readers seem most likely to encounter in clinical practice. Specifically omitted is any discussion of spells, hexes, and possession—topics that are beyond our scope but that may limit the usefulness of this book in cultures in which medical practitioners frequently encounter them. Readers should understand that the perspectives presented do not represent an attempt at consensus and in fact at times sharply disagree with each other. Because clinicians will encounter it, especially if they work with children, we have included Christian Science, a worldview that is at odds with evidence-based medical consensus.

Part III presents implications and applications of the differences among worldviews. The authors of Chapter 12 offer contrasting views on several issues at the nexus of spirituality, ethics, and professionalism. These include the nature of the physician's role and its boundaries, conscientious refusal of care, and the therapeutic use of spiritual interventions. In Chapter 13, Terry Bard and Walter Moczynski, each of whom has directed a hospital department of pastoral care, discuss the evolution of hospital chaplaincy and the contemporary role of the chaplain as a member of the clinical team. In the final chapter, Marta Herschkopf, a student who took our course during her first year of medical school, explores learning and teaching about spirituality in the light of recent developments in medical education.

Inviting physicians who were taking graduate degrees in public health as well as divinity school students as participants and contributors has greatly enriched our course and this book. We hope that this book, while focused on the practical importance of spirituality in medicine, will prove useful to a wider audience of caregivers, patients, and leaders of health care delivery systems.

Many students and several patients deserve thanks for enriching discussions in the course from which this book grew. We are also grateful to Nancy Kehoe and Ed Lowenstein for their experienced perspectives, to Jean Peteet and Meg D'Ambra for their cheerful encouragement, and to Nancy Axelrod for her unerring administrative guidance.

PART I / Historical and Clinical Context

CHAPTER ONE

Spirituality and Biomedicine

A History of Harmony and Discord

Michael J. Balboni, M.Div., Th.M., Ph.D.,
and Tracy A. Balboni, M.D., M.P.H.

In the 1642 treatise *Religio Medici* (The Religion of a Doctor), the English physician Sir Thomas Browne remarked on the public acceptance of the medieval proverb "Tres medici, duo athei" (Where there are three physicians, there are two atheists). He reflected on the belief that study of the natural world and secondary causes turned "the devotion of many unto atheism" (Greenhill 1898, p. 34). Browne suggested that both faith and reason have their own "sovereignty and prerogative in a due time and place," coming under God, who is "the Cause of all."

Browne is one of many physicians who has thoughtfully synthesized belief in God with the study and practice of medicine. But does Browne's argument undermine the medieval proverb or prove its validity? Is the practice of medicine congruent with a spiritual worldview, or does it lead to irreligion? The relationship between medicine and spirituality, like that between science and religion, is not subject to a simple account (Wilson 2002). Its history has been marked by harmony but also punctuated by seasons of suspicion and discord. In this chapter we offer a general historical overview and then consider current questions facing the soul of medicine, particularly in relation to research and clinical practice in the United States.

Our goal is to recount the history of the relationship between spirituality and biomedicine, and also the implications of this history for the practice of medicine today. Our historical review has limitations worth noting at the outset. First, its focus is on the relationship of Western scientific medicine, or biomedicine, to North American and European culture and traditions, primarily Judaism and Christianity (Porter 1994). Other healing traditions, such as Shamanism, Islamic folk medicines, traditional Chinese medicine, and Ayurvedic or Indian medicine, also represent centuries of reflection on the relationship between spiritual practice, psychology, and religion but they will be only peripherally addressed here. A second limitation is that this will be an overview, not a comprehensive academic account.

Harmony: Spirituality as the Healing Narrative

Healing and spirituality have a long-standing interrelationship both conceptually and institutionally. On the conceptual level, the ability to address and heal a person's physical pain and suffering serves as a sign of that spiritual worldview's authenticity and power. Spiritual worldviews also provide a conceptual framework for understanding why a particular person may be physically suffering and how that suffering relates to the spiritual world. Most major religions have viewed the spiritual and the material as inseparable, organically related entities.

On an institutional level, most spiritual worldviews generate practices that attempt to ameliorate physical suffering. Nearly every traditional society has combined the role of healer and priest. One renowned medical historian called this "a strange belief which has persisted through the centuries and millennia with incredible tenacity" (Sigerist 1951, p. 134). This interconnection has also frequently resulted in the use of buildings and other forms of physical space (e.g., monasteries) for the combined aims of spiritual and physical healing. The spiritual worldview has provided not only a larger explanatory model in which illness and healing could be understood but also the context and expertise in which physical healing could occur.

The prevalent and persisting phenomenon of shamanism illustrates the supernatural framework that traditional societies have adopted in understanding disease and healing. The shaman functions as a medium between individuals and a sometimes hostile spiritual world that can be pacified through an array of medical and ritualistic practices to "avoid conflict and sickness as well as ensure fertility" (Risse 1997, p. 49). Though shamans embrace a largely spiritual understanding of illness, they also practice materially focused procedures (e.g., bone setting) and pharmacologic interventions based on empirical experience. This led historian Roy Porter to suggest that there may be unrecognized similarities between contemporary Western medicine and traditional concepts of sickness. Cultural anthropologists also compare the shamanistic use of powerful medicinal remedies with the rituals, beliefs, and structures of biomedicine (Porter 2001).

The connection of the Hippocratic tradition with spiritual devotion to the Asclepian cult is another example of the historic alliance between spirituality and medicine. As distinct from shamanistic folk medicine, Hippocratic medicine is grounded in a natural theory of health and disease. The Hippocratic tradition conceptualizes the physical and emotional qualities of the human being as composed of four humors (blood, phlegm, yellow bile, and black bile), fluidlike substances that in health are properly proportioned. Illness results from humoral excess or deficiency, leading to therapies that aimed to restore balance. But the tradition's naturalism should not be equated with irreligion. Rather, its naturalism was a form of pagan belief in which divinity was immanent with nature. Furthermore, the tradition itself was laden with a "religious aura" (Temkin 1991, p. 191). For example, from its inception, Hippocratic medicine was connected to the healing cult of Asclepius, a cult based on worship of the Greek god of medicine, Asclepius, that rose in Hellenism and persisted at least through the fifth century CE (Edelstein and Edelstein 1998).

The connection of Hippocratic medicine with the religion of the ancient Greeks—highlighted in Asclepian devotion—is illustrated by the Hippocratic Oath. This oath, pledged by early Greek physicians and persisting in modified form into recent medical practice, is founded on a vow to the Greek gods: "I swear by Apollo the physician, and Asclepius, and Hygieia and Panacea and all the gods and goddesses as my witnesses, that, according to my ability and judgment, I will keep this Oath and this contract." Greek physicians' connection with the cult of Asclepius was not simply a "half-hearted concession" (Heynick 2002, p. 53); rather, Hippocratic physicians believed in the power of Asclepius and concluded that he was healer par excellence (Temkin 1991, p. 187).

Asclepius was believed to appear in night visions to supplicants sleeping in the temple (a practice known as incubation). Asclepius would occasionally perform instantaneous miracles; however, most patients received detailed instructions in their dreams regarding those medical procedures that would result in cure. Patients would subsequently turn to their physicians to carry out the god's recommendations. While Asclepius's advice would occasionally break with Hippocratic norms, causing tension with the physicians, the therapies typically complied with up-to-date Hippocratic practices (Edelstein and Edelstein 1998). The relationship between Hippocratic medical practice and Asclepian cultic ritual demonstrates how even a naturalistic approach to medicine included a carefully constructed social and theological alliance with spiritual beliefs and institutions.

While most healing traditions have been formed in alliance with a spiritual worldview, Hippocratic medicine has been unique in that it is a theory and a practice that has been easily reframed and adopted by various spiritual worldviews. This flexibility was essential for a positive embrace by the monotheistic communities of Judaism, Christianity, and later, Islam. Judaism's encounter with shamanistic medicine engendered disapproval of physicians in the Hebrew Bible (2 Chronicles 16:12) because of its alliance with spiritual mediums and magical remedies (Brown 1995).

In contrast, Judaism's encounter with the Hippocratic tradition led to a new posture toward medical practice because its philosophy was easily synthesized with monotheistic beliefs (Jakobovits 1975) that emphasized an axiomatic distinction between Creator and creature and that gave exclusive credit for healing to Yahweh (Exodus 15.26). Because the Hippocratic concept of health and healing is grounded in material as opposed to spiritual realities, it could easily be conceptualized as part of the material world created by God. Similarly, healing practices associated with Hippocratic medicine could be understood as putting into practice the understanding of God's ordered material world to bring about health—a gift to humankind for which God alone deserved credit as the author of that created order. This new context led Ben Sira, writing around the second century BCE, to instruct his Jewish readers to "make friends with the physician for . . . him also God has established in his profession" (Skehan and Di Lella 1987, 38.1). Reflecting a continued spiritual foundation for health and healing despite adopting the materially based principles of Hippocratic medicine, Jewish culture saw the purpose of physical health and healing as serving the spiritual end of knowing God (Dorff 1986).

Christian integration of Hippocratic medicine followed a somewhat different course. By the time Christian communities had developed enough to include organized care for the sick in the third and fourth centuries BCE (Ferngren 1992), Hippocratic medicine was more firmly affixed to the cult of Asclepias than when Jewish peoples encountered it centuries before. Christians rejected the Asclepian healing rite because Jesus and Asclepius could not both be venerated as "Savior" and "Great Physician" (Edelstein and Edelstein 1998). However, when state persecution ceased, the Christian church did employ Hippocratic medicine as an agent of its mission of compassion for the sick (Matthew 25:34–40). Beginning in the fourth and fifth centuries, the church's caring mission led monastic communities in both the East and the West to establish hospitals of care and cure (Miller 1985). Monks became proficient in copying and extending medical texts, and some became skilled physicians advancing medical knowledge. The Rule of St. Benedict, written in the sixth century as a practical guide to Christian communities, made it incumbent upon its ascetic members to "take the greatest care of the sick." The result was a remarkable alliance that "went beyond anything that the classical world had to offer: institutional health care administered in a spirit of compassion by those whose desire to serve God summoned them to a life of active beneficence" (Ferngren 2009, p. 152).

One of the most influential and theologically detailed Christian engagements with Hippocratic medicine came from Basil of Caesarea (d. 379). Basil was a trained Hippocratic practitioner but apparently refused the Hippocratic oath because of its pledge to gods besides Christ (Temkin 1991). After becoming archbishop, he founded what some consider the first hospital on the outskirts of Caesarea (in modern-day Turkey)—described triumphantly as the "new city" because it modeled the highest ideals for a church-governed institution (Miller 1985). Basil asserted that Christians are permitted to practice and receive the benefits of the art of medicine because it was created by God. God's healing power was understood as present in both the material means of medicine and divine intervention. However, Basil warned in his Long Rules (55) that physical health and healing should not be pursued to the extent that it "turns our whole life into one long provision for the flesh" (Silvas 2005).

In Basil's view, physical health and healing were secondary, subject to the primary good of spiritual salvation. He taught that medicine served as a "pattern for the healing of the soul" (Silvas 2005), so medicine and physical healing were beneficial only when they directly served the goal of eternal salvation. In Basil's understanding, disease and healing provided a physical picture or "pattern" for comprehending and experiencing spiritual truths. When medicine for the body was practiced in such a way as to teach a person about spiritual needs, it served a higher purpose. However, when medicine was practiced or received in a way disconnected from the spiritual truths to which they intrinsically pointed as signs, Basil taught that medicine was "worthy of cattle" because it served no spiritual purpose. For Basil, Hippocratic medicine could be rightly understood only as it pointed to the story of the Bible culminating in Jesus Christ. Recognized as one of the great teachers of the church, Basil established an influential synthesis of medicine and Christian theology that shaped a Christian understanding of the medical profession into early modern times.

Those who held dual roles as physicians and clerics in Islamic, Jewish, and Christian communities further illustrate a medical-spiritual synthesis. This was a widespread practice throughout medieval Europe (Amundsen 1986). Kealey estimated that at least 38 percent of physicians in medieval England were monks or priests (1981, p. 40). The prominent physician-rabbi Moses Maimonides reflects a similar phenomenon. The Prayer of Maimonides, falsely attributed to Maimonides (Rosner 1998), provides a compelling 18th-century portrait of the way in which Jewish faith informs medical practice as a divine vocation. The physician prays to rely on God because "without Thy help not even the least thing will succeed" (Freeman and Abrams 1999, p. 161). The prayer interpreted sickness in the light of the providence of God, who "sendest to man diseases as beneficent messengers to foretell approaching danger and to urge him to avert it." This religious interpretation of the meaning of illness also spurred some Jewish physicians to encourage the sufferer "to ask God's forgiveness through prayer and fasting" (Ruderman 1988, p. 33). For Maimonides, not unlike Basil, bodily sickness and health were both secondary goods ordered on behalf of the spiritual life. The physician's vocation of aiming for physical health was not a good unto itself but was, according to Maimonides, "in order that his soul be upright to know the Lord" (Rosner 1979, p. 53).

Physician-clerics were widespread in 17th-century New England in what one scholar described as a widespread "angelical conjunction" (Watson 1991). Like Maimonides, they often offered unique perspectives on how religious traditions shape the goals and practices of a medical vocation. An eminent English Puritan pastor-physician, Richard Baxter (d. 1691), gave extended instructions regarding the "the duty of physicians," cautioning physicians not to pursue wealth, always to help the poor, and to yield to better physicians with humility. Baxter also exhorted physicians to "depend on God for your direction and success." To avoid missing a diagnosis or incorrectly performing a procedure, he advised the physician to "earnestly crave [God's] help and blessing." He also taught that caring for the sick and dying, rather than leading to a physician's "hardened heart," should engender deeper spirituality and cause physicians to be "more industrious in preparing for the life to come" (Baxter 1673, p. 111). This meant for Baxter that physicians should care for patients' souls, and not only their physical bodies. Physicians have a unique opportunity to speak "a few serious words" (p. 114) about salvation and judgment—an opportunity some pastors may not be afforded. "Think not to excuse yourselves by saying, 'It is the pastor's duty.' For though it be theirs ex officio, it is yours also ex charitate. Charity bindeth every man, as he hath opportunity, to do good to all, and especially the greatest good" (p. 113). In Baxter's understanding, sickness arouses spiritual needs and questions, and faithful physicians must address them by using their power and position out of love for souls. Echoing the prioritization of spiritual over physical matters seen in many medical-spiritual symbioses of the past, physical cure is ordered by Baxter as ancillary to the spiritual healing of souls.

This brief and selective survey suggests that the relationship between medicine and spirituality has been largely harmonious and interdependent (Porter 1994). Because sickness and healing have been interpreted as spiritual events across cultures, ages, and religions, healers have been viewed as allies and conduits of spiritual powers. This is evident not only in folk medicine but also in Hippocratic and early Western biomedicine. Though with different emphases and practices for disparate healing traditions, spirituality has provided an overall interpretive framework for the experience of sickness and the practice of medicine.

Discord: Ironies of Medicine and Spiritual Communities

While it is clear that most physicians have not worn the garments of irreligion, the fabric of the historic alliance between medicine and spirituality has in more recent times been torn apart for a number of theological and sociological reasons. Contemporary definitions of medicine likely reflect and reinforce this divide. We define biomedicine as an approach to health and healing shaped by four rational principles: (1) materialism, which has led to a mind-body dualism; (2) reductionism, which has led to an ontological understanding of the origin of disease; (3) empiricism, which has emphasized numerical measurements and probabilistic reasoning (Risse 1997); and (4) the objectivity of physicians whose role does not include innate, therapeutic ability. Ironically, this scientific approach to health and healing grew from and has been primarily nurtured by cultures influenced by Jewish and Christian presuppositions. In this section we consider five historical developments fostering the separation of medicine and spirituality. The events discussed below are not the only ones that produced this rift, but they were catalytic or were milestone events in a process of divergence.

The Fourth Lateran Council

One of the most influential medieval reforms affecting the relationship of the Christian church to Western medicine came in 1215 from the Fourth Lateran Council. Historians generally understand this council to have secured and tightened the exercise of papal influence over church and society. Canon 22 declared that "physicians of the body called to the bedside of the sick shall before all advise them to call for the physician of souls, so that, spiritual health being restored, bodily health will follow" (www.fordham.edu/halsall/basis/lateran4.html). This canon also asserted the primacy of the soul over the body, a potential causal relationship between moral sin and physical sickness, and the professional responsibility of physicians to coordinate their efforts with care of souls. In this way, the canon ensures that the confession of sins be included in the care of the sick—no matter how serious or trivial the ailment. Additionally, making confession a regular component of medical care was intended to prevent the sick person from assuming that the offering of confession meant immanent death (Amundsen 1986). Physicians were to invite the sick to confess their sins to a priest before an initial medical examination in order to stem this worry.

On one hand, this canon serves as an important example of the concord between the medical profession and church authorities. Physicians of the body were to work together with physicians of the soul by recognizing the potential spiritual source for sickness and by encouraging repentance as the first order of response. On the other hand, the canon also marks an important ecclesiastical decision institutionalizing a division of labor, demarcating matters of the body from matters of the soul. While such a division was not strange in practice, it was new on the level of an ecclesiastical formalization.

This can be contrasted with the situation of several hundred years earlier, when Basil of Caesarea had applauded the physician Eustathius for "not confining the application of your skill to men's bodies, but by attending also to the cure of the diseases of their souls" (Basil of Caesarea, letter 189). The Fourth Lateran Council, in contrast, expects cooperation from physicians on spiritual matters but no direct spiritual intervention, at least in regard to confession. The primary motivation behind this ruling was not practical—to establish a division of labor between priests and physicians—but to reestablish papal authority over the social and intellectual milieu of European culture, which had been waning during the late 12th century, as well as to combat doctrinal challenges from heretical groups advocating antisacerdotal beliefs (Cantor 1994). Mandating that only priests receive confession heightened the importance of priestly authority and, consequently, furthered the church's ability to exercise direct supervision over the beliefs and lives of the laity. This ruling, combined with similar ecclesiastical rulings of the 12th and 13th centuries that limited the practice of clerical medicine (Amundsen 1996), had the unintended consequence, however, of eroding the vocational influence of clergy on the practice of medicine. As a result, during the 13th century large portions of Europe saw a significant demographic shift from clerics to secular physicians (Ziegler 1998)—trained in universities rather than monasteries—so in France during 1300–1345, only 1 percent of physicians were also clerics (McVaugh 1993). The 13th century marks an emerging divide between spirituality and medicine (Ziegler 1998).

The Reformation

A second key historical event in the Christian tradition influencing the relationship of spiritual communities to medicine was the Protestant Reformation, which began in 1517. Societies that adopted the philosophies of the Protestant Reformation made religious and political decisions that had unintended consequences for how religion and medical care would relate in its aftermath. Reformation policies, based on an anticlericalism that regarded the misuse of donated funds and abuse of power among clergy and religious orders as an entrenched evil (McGrath 1993), sought to dissolve rather than reform monastic houses. Legislation closed many monasteries and religious houses in Protestant districts. While these enactments did not directly target hospitals, many of them were also closed because most were part of larger religious orders (Orme and Webster 1995). Protestants did attempt to erect hospitals to care for the infirm and poor, as can be seen in the legislative actions of Luther (Lindberg 1986) and Calvin (Smylie 1986). However, their approach differed from the medieval Christian approach to health care; because Protestants rejected ties with church institutions perceived as corrupt, these hospitals lacked sufficient centralized power and infrastructure to fully support the increasingly complex care of sick persons. The only centralized power remaining that could provide this infrastructure resided in the state; hence, Protestant hospitals relied on close alliances with governments for financial support. Ecclesiastical influences on hospitals waned further as the ideology of separation between church and state slowly took root during the Enlightenment.

While Roman Catholic provinces continued to show strong support for public health charities, there was a noticeable wane under Protestant influence. Amanda Porterfield (2005) argued that Reformation spirituality brought a new emphasis on self-analytical, individualized piety, which diminished energy that may have given public expression in Christian health care. With a strong emphasis on spiritual self-analysis and a rejection of works salvation, there was less need, she argues, for visible demonstration of public works. In its place was a heightened emphasis on home health care manuals and herbal remedies, supported by a Protestant commitment to the "home as a center for religious life" and female homemakers' serving as the primary caregivers to the sick. While this model may have compensated somewhat for the loss of hospitals and provided a potentially strong emphasis on spiritual care, it also led to a diminished emphasis on hospitals and the medical profession. When medical care later moved back to a specialization model because of medical advancements, responsibilities associated with spiritual care were no longer considered essential to the medical profession.

The Protestant Reformation also disrupted the long-standing relationship between physicians and religious orders. With the dissolution of monastic life in Protestant Europe, the medical profession would no longer receive physicians who carried explicit religious vows. Instead, the Reformation emphasized the holiness and divine calling in "worldly business" (Placher 2005, p. 412). However, with the rise of such Enlightenment philosophies as Descartes' dualism (1637), emphasizing a dichotomy between matters of the mind and of the body, spiritual matters such as "divine calling" were increasingly considered separate from material matters. The developing "Protestant work ethic" limited one's spiritual calling in work to one's personal motivation and approach (e.g., honesty and hard work). This transformed the robust religious identity of many physicians into an internalized spirituality that upheld virtues important to personal motivation (e.g., integrity) but did not permit direct engagement of spiritual matters raised by healing and illness (Weber, Baehr, and Wells 2002). Thus, the Reformation set the stage for a loss of religious identity among physicians and undercut spiritually informed modes of care by the medical profession. This process would accelerate in later centuries.

Enlightenment: The Mechanization of the Body

A third key contributor to the extant gulf between spirituality and medicine was the development of scientific medicine during the 17th and 18th centuries. The rise of science led to a dramatic shift in attitudes toward authority, epistemology, and theological anthropology that reshaped the medical profession (Cunningham and French 1990). The Enlightenment age brought fresh optimism that scientific medicine could, in the words of Francis Bacon (d. 1626), bring "relief of man's estate." This hope eventually developed for some into a quasi-religious belief that medical science could bring about "human emancipation, ensuring freedom from suffering, want, and fear" (Conrad et al. 1995, p. 374). With the promise of scientific medicine to bring freedom from suffering came a strong disdain for ancient authorities viewed as hampering scientific progress, including ecclesiastical, biblical, and Galenic (Hippocratic) medicine. Scientifically based medicine depended on observation and validation through experimentation. Newton's discovery of the physical laws of cause and effect promoted the reductionistic belief that all complex phenomena can be explained in terms of their summative parts. The Enlightenment's dualistic anthropology led to a conception of the human body as principally a machine. Together, these philosophies of the new scientific medicine led to a slow but critical shift in the focus, aims, and felt responsibilities of physicians.

The Enlightenment did not necessarily breed disdain among physicians toward religion (Grell and Cunningham 2007). Rather, it further propelled the profession as a whole into a dualistic conception of the relationship between body and soul. Spirituality—as the expression of the immaterial reality of humanity—became secondary in a profession primarily concerned with material matters and means of addressing them. Ironically, many who adopted dualism during this time did not therefore accept materialism; instead, they chose to believe in the immortality of the soul and the absolute necessity of an "immaterial principle" (Wright 2000, pp. 253–54). Many key figures involved in the philosophical shifts of the Enlightenment period were devoutly religious; these included Francis Bacon, René Descartes, and Isaac Newton. In reflecting on the motivations of 17th-century mechanical philosophers, the medical historian Lawrence

Conrad writes that for them, "God was still at the centre of their enterprise, for they were intent on revealing the laws and workmanship of God in order to praise Him and to confirm His existence" (Conrad et al. 1995, p. 345). Nevertheless, as physicians became more scientifically oriented, they became focused on cure rather than care (Risse 1999). The social and functional implications of their new philosophy left little basis for addressing the spiritual dimensions of the practice of medicine or their patients' experience of illness.

"Physician Scientists"

A fourth important contributor to the schism between spiritual expression and the practice of medicine was a carefully orchestrated identification between physicians and science, the roots of which can be traced at least to the Enlightenment (Risse 1986). As Paul Starr explains, the rise of medical authority and the establishment of the profession as a healing authority are due in large measure to the fact that medical practitioners consciously presented themselves to an American public as engaged in a scientific enterprise (Starr 1982). Through such a connection, physicians were able to differentiate themselves from others who were portrayed (perhaps accurately at times) as quacks offering inferior therapies. They were also able to create a professional monopoly over the prescribing of medication, eligibility for state-funded research, and reimbursements for patient care.

Aligning medicine with science was not the sole reason for the emergence of the profession of medicine during the 19th century in the United States. Sociologist Jonathan Imber (2008) points out that physicians were also allied with Protestantism and physicians during this time. He argues that Protestant clergy empowered the medical profession with a moral and spiritual vocation, resulting in a deeply held public trust of physicians. This trust was grounded not merely in the scientific competence of doctors, but also in their moral character and spiritual credibility. From Imber's analysis, one could conclude that present-day public trust in the profession has declined in part because these spiritual roots no longer authorize it. The profession currently has only its scientific credentials remaining.

What is less clear about the 19th- to 20th-century alliance between medicine and science is how much it may have catalyzed the distancing of the medical profession from spiritual and moral concerns. We suggest here three possible, and potentially overlapping, hypotheses requiring further historical and sociological research. First, in the popular American imagination, there has been a persistent perception of conflict between science and religion. Because physicians have been viewed as on the side of science, they may have come to be seen as less than open to mixing these domains. A second hypothesis is that scientific objectivity may have come to be seen as incompatible with religious subjectivity. Since the time of Immanuel Kant, religion has been widely perceived to be a domain of subjective, internal values separate from the domain of empirical phenomena. Seeing themselves as on the side of science, physicians have sometimes eschewed subjectivity so as not to be misled by it in the search to establish the underlying material causes of disease. They have come to regard practice as ideally evidence-based. A third hypothesis is that scientifically oriented physicians may have come to apply rational rules appropriate for public discourse (Habermas 1989) to what is a private relationship with an individual patient. Forces such as pluralism and bureaucratization have altered this relationship to the point where it is commonly experienced as a meeting of two strangers who may not share similar spiritual worldviews. Patients' perceptions of physicians as scientists may precondition both patients and physicians to expect that conversations about health and therapy should be conducted in the languages of science and rationality.

Medical Missions and Catholic Hospitals

The remaining two milestone events in the development of a schism between spirituality and medicine have taken place more recently. Both exemplify a serious engagement of medicine by the Christian tradition, but ironically they have widened the gulf between spirituality and medicine. The first is the Christian medical missions movement. Medical missions enlist Christian medical practitioners to provide medical care to those in need, both as an expression of the healing power of the good news, or gospel (Jansen 1995), and as a practical avenue for sharing that good news (Hardiman 2006). Medical missions offer Christian medical practitioners an arena in which they can more naturally integrate faith and medical work. However, by focusing the Christian calling to care for the sick largely in non-Western contexts, this movement has furthered its absence from secular ones and diverted attention from how that integration might occur in more complex, secular medical settings.

A second important development is the growth and subsequent decline of Roman Catholic hospitals. In the U.S. medical context, Catholics have shown a remarkable ability to bring together spirituality and medicine. By 1885, Catholics had opened 154 U.S. hospitals, nearly doubling the total hospitals available in the United States (Rosenberg 1987). These often addressed the need to care for poor Catholic immigrants who experienced cultural and religious prejudice in a Protestant culture. Supported by the church's hierarchy, religious orders such as the Sisters of Mercy and the Sisters of Charity worked to "institutionalize medical treatment that infused standard medical practice with a Roman Catholic perspective on life and death" (McCauley 2005, p. 1). Their institutional ethos was infused with religious ritual and identity. In many of the hospitals, the sisters "automatically had a position of authority" because of their religious status (Risse 1999, p. 524). At Mercy Hospital in Buffalo, for example, each morning began with the celebration of the Eucharist, and the day was punctuated with prayers over the loudspeaker at 7:00 a.m., noon, 6:00 p.m., and 9:00 p.m. (Risse 1999). Physicians, interns, and nurses were all expected to share the religious worldview and ethical system espoused by the church. Pope Pius XII described these hospitals as "the fairest flowers of missionary endeavor," and another advocate wrote that prayers lent "the art of medicine . . . prestige and dignity" (Risse 1999, pp. 522, 529).

Since the 1960s, however, Catholic hospitals have experienced a crisis of identity and have declined. One reason has been the influence of Medicare, which greatly expanded hospital bureaucracy and forced a shift in institutional goals and methods of decision making. The increasing complexity of medical care also has led to increasing professionalization of medical caregivers, with a greater focus on efficiency and specialization than on caregivers' religious views. As medical historian Guenter Risse (1999) notes, within one generation the emphasis in Catholic hospitals shifted from the aim of experiencing sickness as a spiritual rebirth to the aim of offering highly technological care. A second, and arguably more important, reason for decline was the effect on the identity of Catholic health care providers brought about by Vatican II. In the document *Lumen Gentium*, this council laid new emphasis on the "apostolate of the laity," lifting up common people working in the "world" as God's spirit-filled priests and prophets. Rather than being passive participants of the church, the laity were newly encouraged in their daily work to "impregnate culture and human works with a moral value" with the goal that "the world may be filled with the Spirit of Christ" (IV.36). The church's new emphasis on the role of the laity, however, led to a noticeable drop in initiates choosing monastic life (Risse 1999). Vatican II also reconfigured the leadership of hospitals, moving them from religious orders to Catholic laity. Despite the ideals established by Vatican II, it is also likely that the laity were not yet prepared to offer a conspicuous form of religious leadership as previously experienced under religious orders.

While contemporary Catholic hospitals have maintained a bioethical moral code following religious norms, the culture of ritual and care that once permeated them has waned and is often absent. Here again, religious decisions have led to unintended consequences, separating religious forms of spirituality from medical care. In the judgment of one critic, Roman Catholic health care has been transformed from an institution that once provided care that was "flagrantly Christian" to an organization in which "there is no longer a commitment to embedding all actions in an all-pervasive and particular Christian self-consciousness" (Engelhardt 2000, pp. 380–81).

Is Rapprochement Possible?

While scientific medicine has been understood as the contemporary descendent of Greek medicine because of their shared naturalistic basis, scientific medicine broke from its predecessor by following a reductionistic rather than an integrated approach to health and disease (Porter 1996). This reductionistic model has prompted a series of protests from others attempting to revive holistic views. Recently, protests against fragmentation of the person in the West have taken the form of "alternative" or "complementary" approaches to health and healing that either directly compete with or run in parallel with conventional scientific medicine. All of these espouse a view that "health and sickness involve the whole person—often the whole cosmos" (Porter 1996, p. 113). By virtue of being more congruent with a spiritual philosophy of life than the view found in biomedicine (Astin 1998), alternative medicine has often been fueled by various religious movements and spiritual beliefs, including those led by Paracelsus (16th c.), Mesmer (18th c.), Wesley (18th c.), Swedenborg (18th c.), Hahnemann (19th c.), and Mary Baker Eddy (19th c.). Spiritual worldviews have also fostered faith healing by Pentecostals and Catholics, as well as contemporary New Age approaches characterized by an eclectic array of spiritual practices.

While complementary and alternative medicine (CAM) has only begun to acquire an evidence base, the past few decades have seen a rapidly expanding corpus of literature on the relationship between spirituality and health (Koenig 2008; Koenig, McCullough, and Larson 2001). Like the CAM movement, the spirituality and health movement expresses a yearning for a holistic approach to the healing of persons that overcomes historical and contemporary obstacles to reintegrating spirituality and healing (Sulmasy 2006). Data from scientific studies of the intersection of spirituality, health, and illness have demonstrated a relationship between spirituality and the experience, and at times the outcome, of illness in areas such as quality of life in the face of declining health, medical decision making, and health behaviors (Koenig 2008). The implications of these findings have been controversial (Shuman and Meador 2003; Sloan 2006) in part because, as a protest against reductionistic medicine, the spirituality and health movement has borrowed the methods and language of biomedicine for validation. Given the body of data supporting a central role of spirituality in the experience of illness, national organizations are increasingly including spirituality when setting standards of good-quality medical care (Joint Commission 2008; NCP 2009; NICE 2004; WHO 2004). Despite these developments, clinicians only infrequently recognize patients' spiritual concerns (Balboni et al. 2007).

While the future direction of the relationship between spirituality and biomedicine remains unknown, this brief overview underscores the long-standing and intimate relationship that religion and spirituality have shared with the medical profession and its care of the sick. In particular, religious communities have held an important role in both establishing and diminishing the relationship between spirituality and medicine. A reemergence of the voices and presence of religious communities in the practice of medicine, both clergy and laity, will be an important factor in any rehemming of a once-seamless garment. Some may caution against reintroducing religious communities and theological traditions into the practice of medicine. Others advocate for definitions and understandings of spirituality as distinct from religion, motivated in part by a desire to be inclusive of varieties of experiences and worldviews. Particular religious communities, in contrast, may be reluctant to minimize distinct beliefs and practices that seem to them essential features of their tradition. In the midst of these differing concerns, a sizable majority of the U.S. population expresses a desire for medical care providers to take spirituality into better account by (Astrow and Sulmasy 2004). The ability of leaders in the spirituality and health movement to go beyond protest to build consensus on complex and pressing questions is likely to determine the movement's sustainability and impact.

Consider in conclusion four choices that seem central to the development of a widely disseminated, sustainable model of spiritually respectful, inclusive, and effective care.

1. *Complementary versus assimilated.* Should the medical system cooperate with representatives of spirituality and religion while maintaining a division of labor, or should spirituality be more completely integrated throughout the medical system as a core component and context for health and healing?
2. *Functional versus substantive.* Should spiritual practices be evaluated and promoted primarily on the grounds that they may have salutary effects on the body and mind, or should spiritual practices be embraced irrespective of their physical and mental effects, based instead on their theological and spiritual merits?
3. *Generic versus tradition-constituted.* Should spirituality research and spiritual care be grounded primarily in a theory of our basic humanity, autonomous of theological tradition, or is the nature of spirituality and spiritual care intrinsically informed by religious communities, theological methods, and tradition-constituted stories and language?
4. *Pluralism versus particular communities.* What role should particular religious communities play in a spiritually charged but irreducibly pluralistic context such as Western medicine? Should the medical profession foster and encourage the presence of particular religious communities in caring for the sick? What role should religious communities assume in shaping the vocational calling, moral practices, and spiritual care of clinicians generally and in the lives of those health professionals who are members of religious communities?

Thoughtful dialogue among representatives of medical, spiritual, and humanistic traditions will be important in formulating the answers to these questions and shaping the future direction of their relationship.

REFERENCES

Amundsen, D. W. 1986. The medieval Catholic tradition. In *Caring and Curing: Health and Medicine in the Western Religious Tradition*, ed. R. L. Numbers and D. W. Amundsen. Baltimore: Johns Hopkins University Press.

———. 1996. *Medicine, Society, and Faith in the Ancient and Medieval Worlds*. Baltimore: Johns Hopkins University Press.

Astin, J. A. 1998. Why patients use alternative medicine: Results of a national study. *JAMA* 279 (19): 1548–53.

Astrow, A. B., and D. P. Sulmasy. 2004. Spirituality and the patient-physician relationship. *JAMA* 291 (23): 2884.

Balboni, T. A., L. C. Vanderwerker, S. D. Block, M. E. Paulk, C. S. Lathan, J. R. Peteet, and H. G. Prigerson. 2007. Religiousness and spiritual support among advanced cancer patients and associations with end-of-life treatment preferences and quality of life. *Journal of Clinical Oncology* 25 (5): 555–60.

Baxter, R. 1673. *A Christian Directory: or, A Summ of Practical Theologie, and Cases of Conscience, Directing Christians, How to Use Their Knowledge and Faith*. London: Printed by Robert White, for Nevill Simmons.

Brown, M. L. 1995. *Israel's Divine Healer*. Grand Rapids, MI: Zondervan.

Cantor, N. F. 1994. *The Civilization of the Middle Ages*. New York: HarperPerennial.

Conrad, L. I., M. Neve, V. Nutton, R. Porter, and A. Wear. 1995. *The Western Medical Tradition, 800 B.C.–1800 A.D.* Cambridge: Cambridge University Press.

Cunningham, A., and R. K. French. 1990. *The Medical Enlightenment of the Eighteenth Century*. Cambridge: Cambridge University Press.

Dorff, E. 1986. The Jewish tradition. In *Caring and Curing: Health and Medicine in the Western Religious Traditions*, ed. R. L. Numbers and D. W. Amundsen. Baltimore: Johns Hopkins University Press.

Edelstein, E. J., and L. Edelstein. 1998. *Asclepius: A Collection and Interpretation of the Testimonies*. Baltimore: Johns Hopkins University Press.

Engelhardt, H. T. 2000. *The Foundations of Christian Bioethics*. Lisse, The Netherlands: Swets & Zeitlinger.

Ferngren, G. B. 1992. Early Christianity as a religion of healing. *Bulletin of the History of Medicine* 66 (1): 1–15.

———. 2009. *Medicine and Health Care in Early Christianity*. Baltimore: Johns Hopkins University Press.

Freeman, D. L., and J. Z. Abrams. 1999. *Illness and Health in the Jewish Tradition: Writings from the Bible to Today*. Philadelphia: Jewish Publication Society.

Greenhill, W. A. 1898. *Sir Thomas Browne's "Religio Medici."* New York: Macmillan.

Grell, O. P., and A. Cunningham. 2007. *Medicine and Religion in Enlightenment Europe: The History of Medicine in Context*. Aldershot, Eng.: Ashgate.

Habermas, J. 1989. *The Structural Transformation of the Public Sphere: An Inquiry into a Category of Bourgeois Society*. Studies in Contemporary German Social Thought. Cambridge: MIT Press.

Hardiman, D. 2006. *Healing Bodies, Saving Souls: Medical Missions in Asia and Africa.* Amsterdam: Rodopi.

Heynick, F. 2002. *Jews and Medicine: An Epic Saga*. Hoboken, NJ: KTAV Publishing.

Imber, J. B. 2008. *Trusting Doctors: The Decline of Moral Authority in American Medicine*. Princeton: Princeton University Press.

Jakobovits, I. 1975. *Jewish Medical Ethics: A Comparative and Historical Study of the Jewish Religious Attitude to Medicine and Its Practice*. New York: Bloch Publishing.

Jansen, G. 1995. Christian ministry of healing on its way to the year 2000: An archeology of medical missions. *Missiology* 23 (3): 295–307.

Joint Commission. 2008. *Provision of Care, Treatment, and Services: Spiritual Assessment.* The Joint Commission, 2008. www.jointcommission.org/AccreditationPrograms/LongTermCare/Standards/09_FAQs/PC/Spiritual_Assessment.htm. Accessed 15 May 2009.

Kealey, E. J. 1981. *Medieval Medicus: A Social History of Anglo-Norman Medicine*. Baltimore: Johns Hopkins University Press.

Koenig, H. G. 2008. *Medicine, Religion, and Health: Where Science and Spirituality Meet*. West Conshohocken, PA: Templeton Foundation Press.

Koenig, H. G., M. E. McCullough, and D. B. Larson. 2001. *Handbook of Religion and Health*. New York: Oxford University Press.

Lindberg, C. 1986. The Lutheran tradition. In *Caring and Curing: Health and Medicine in the Western Religious Traditions*, ed. R. L. Numbers and D. W. Amundsen. Baltimore: Johns Hopkins University Press.

McCauley, B. 2005. *Who Shall Take Care of Our Sick? Roman Catholic Sisters and the Development of Catholic Hospitals in New York City*. Baltimore: Johns Hopkins University Press.

McGrath, A. E. 1993. *Reformation Thought: An Introduction*. 2nd ed. Oxford: Blackwell.

McVaugh, M. R. 1993. *Medicine before the Plague: Practitioners and Their Patients in the Crown of Aragon, 1285–1345*. New York: Cambridge University Press.

Miller, T. S. 1985. The birth of the hospital in the Byzantine Empire. *Henry E Sigerist Supplemental Bulletin of the History of Medicine*, no. 10, 1–288.

NCP (National Consensus Project for Quality Palliative Care). 2009. *Clinical Practice Guidelines for Quality Palliative Care*. 2nd ed. National Consensus Project, 2009. www.nationalconsensusproject.org/guideline.pdf. Accessed 15 May 2009.

NICE (National Institute for Clinical Excellence). 2004. *Improving Supportive and Palliative Care for Adults with Cancer: The Manual*. National Institute for Clinical Excellence, 2004. www.nice.org.uk/nicemedia/pdf/csgspmanual.pdf. Accessed 15 May 2009.

Orme, N., and M. E. Graham Webster. 1995. *The English Hospital, 1070–1570*. New Haven: Yale University Press.

Placher, W. C. 2005. *Callings: Twenty Centuries of Christian Wisdom on Vocation*. Grand Rapids: Eerdmans.

Porter, R. 1994. Religion and medicine. In *Companion Encyclopedia of the History of Medicine*, ed. W. F. Bynum and R. Porter. New York: Routledge.

———, ed. 1996. *The Cambridge Illustrated History of Medicine*. Cambridge: Cambridge University Press.

———. 2001. What is disease? In *The Cambridge Illustrated History of Medicine*, ed. R. Porter. Cambridge: Cambridge University Press.

Porterfield, A. 2005. *Healing in the History of Christianity*. Oxford: Oxford University Press.

Risse, G. B. 1986. *Hospital Life in Enlightenment Scotland: Care and Teaching at the Royal Infirmary of Edinburgh*. Cambridge: Cambridge University Press.

———. 1997. Medical care. In *Companion Encyclopedia of the History of Medicine*, ed. W. F. Bynum and R. Porter. London: Routledge.

———. 1999. *Mending Bodies, Saving Souls: A History of Hospitals*. New York: Oxford University Press.

Rosenberg, C. E. 1987. *The Care of Strangers: The Rise of America's Hospital System*. New York: Basic Books.

Rosner, F. 1979. The physician and the patient in Jewish law. In *Jewish Bioethics*, ed. F. Rosner, J. D. Bleich, and M. M. Brayer. New York: Sanhedrin Press.

———. 1998. *The Medical Legacy of Moses Maimonides*. Hoboken, NJ: KTAV Publishing.

Ruderman, D. B. 1988. *Kabbalah, Magic, and Science: The Cultural Universe of a Sixteenth-Century Jewish physician*. Cambridge: Harvard University Press.
Shuman, J. J., and K. G. Meador. 2003. *Heal Thyself: Spirituality, Medicine, and the Distortion of Christianity*. New York: Oxford University Press.
Sigerist, H. E. 1951. *A History of Medicine*. New York: Oxford University Press.
Silvas, A. 2005. *The Asketikon of St. Basil the Great*. Oxford: Oxford University Press.
Skehan, P. W., and A. A. Di Lella. 1987. *The Wisdom of Ben Sira: A New Translation with Notes*. Garden City, NY: Doubleday.
Sloan, R. P. 2006. *Blind Faith: The Unholy Alliance of Religion and Medicine*. New York: St. Martin's.
Smylie, J. 1986. The reformed tradition. In *Caring and Curing: Health and Medicine in the Western Religious Traditions*, ed. R. L. Numbers and D. W. Amundsen. Baltimore: Johns Hopkins University Press.
Starr, P. 1982. *The Social Transformation of American Medicine*. New York: Basic Books.
Sulmasy, D. P. 2006. *The Rebirth of the Clinic: An Introduction to Spirituality in Health Care*. Washington, DC: Georgetown University Press.
Temkin, O. 1991. *Hippocrates in a World of Pagans and Christians*. Baltimore: Johns Hopkins University Press.
Watson, P. A. 1991. *The Angelical Conjunction: The Preacher-Physicians of Colonial New England*. Knoxville: University of Tennessee Press.
Weber, M., P. R. Baehr, and G. C. Wells. 2002. *The Protestant Ethic and the "Spirit" of Capitalism and Other Writings*. New York: Penguin Books.
WHO (World Health Organization). 2004. *Palliative Care: Symptom Management and End of Life Care; Integrated Management of Adolescent and Adult Illness*. http://ftp.who.int/htm/IMAI/Modules/IMAI_palliative.pdf. Accessed 15 May 2009.
Wilson, D. B. 2002. The historiography of science and religion. In *Science and Religion: A Historical Introduction*, ed. G. B. Ferngren. Baltimore: Johns Hopkins University Press.
Wright, J. P. 2000. Substance versus function dualism in eighteenth-century medicine. In *Psyche and Soma: Physicians and Metaphysicians on the Mind-Body Problem from Antiquity to Enlightenment*, ed. J. P. Wright and P. Potter. Oxford: Oxford University Press.
Ziegler, J. 1998. *Medicine and Religion, c. 1300: The Case of Arnau de Vilanova*. Oxford: Oxford University Press.

CHAPTER TWO

Approaching Spirituality in Clinical Practice

John R. Peteet, M.D.; Michael J. Balboni, M.Div., Th.M., Ph.D.; and Michael N. D'Ambra, M.D.

A Philosophical Framework: Is the Integration of Faith and Medicine Unethical?

Richard Sloan, an outspoken critic of the "religion, spirituality, and medicine" movement, has argued that the integration of faith and medicine is based on poor science, contributes to the unethical medical practice, and is corrosive of religion (2006). Sloan raises important objections requiring thoughtful dialogue among the medical and religious communities and in society at large. This book is an attempt to continue dialogue about these complex and at times contentious issues.

In our view, many of Sloan's criticisms are valid. For example, many researchers concur with him that the quality of research in spirituality and healing has been lacking. While his criticisms do not apply to all of the research in this field, questions about scientific quality must be taken seriously. Sloan also claims that integrating religion and health care carries the danger of instrumentalizing religion. Using religion for its health benefits obscures the value and importance that it may have in its own right. Others, such as Shuman and

Meador (2003), have demonstrated that turning religious faith into one of the many tools of medicine is theologically naïve. Using religion in this way is inconsistent with many religious claims, resulting in an inappropriate subverting of the ends of religion into bodily health. Respecting others' religious claims, regardless of whether one actually holds to those claims, requires that one not alter the meaning of the claims in order to fit one's own paradigm. Instrumentalizing religion has all too often been the unstated paradigm underlying much research among the psychological disciplines on spirituality and health. Nevertheless, while this is an important caution, the integration of spirituality and health care does not by definition presuppose a functional use of religion. We agree with Sloan that there are important ethical questions to be considered when incorporating religion or spirituality into health care. However, as we note later in this chapter, we see issues such as religious coercion as important cautions rather than insurmountable ethical barriers.

A fundamental issue that is consistently bypassed by many colleagues in discussing these matters is the nature of medicine. How do we understand medicine, health, and disease? What does it mean to provide cure and care? What is a physician? On what authority does one ground one's views? It becomes clear upon reflection that such fundamental questions are difficult to answer. However, it is also clear that medical practice exists within a culture and each culture has a religious or philosophical component. In theological parlance, these components can be expressed as religious or philosophical "norms." Examples of such normative aspects of a culture include (1) basic beliefs or first principles concerning the existence and nature of God or "the other" and (2) basic beliefs concerning the nature and ends of humanity. Norms function authoritatively in that they both guide the community and serve to judge questions confronting the tradition. They are warranted on their own terms within a tradition and are subsequently not empirically verifiable.

Many assume answers to questions about the nature of medicine on the basis of prevailing social constructions, without critical examination. Within given societies, such viewpoints on the meaning of health, disease, care, and cure operate on a normative level but remain untested. Indeed, the more cohesive the society, the less likely that its basic presuppositions will be critically examined. We believe that sweeping criticisms of the spirituality and health movement such as those offered by Sloan suffer (at least in their publication) from inadequate reflection on the nature of medicine and a cluster of related questions.

But what this book attempts to answer is not really the question of whether medicine, religion, and spirituality *should* be related but, rather, *how* that relationship is construed. We assume that one cannot engage basic questions regarding the nature of what medicine itself should be like without heavily resting one's argument on philosophical or theological foundations, which are grounded in traditions. There is a need, as the philosopher Alasdair MacIntyre (1984) has argued, to personally admit, "I find myself part of a history and that is generally to say, whether I like it or not, whether I recognize it or not, one of the bearers of a tradition" (p. 221). Traditions, and the moral communities that embody them, shape the limits, ethics, and goals of medicine. Even those physician scientists who explicitly claim to be free of tradition are in actuality influenced and molded by the Enlightenment tradition of scientific positivism. By claiming freedom from tradition, these physicians are simply expressing a core commitment to their Enlightenment creed. It is a core commitment that on a normative level can be no more privileged than an explicitly theological creed.

Consequently, medicine as a practice is shaped by moral, philosophical, and religious traditions and is embodied by practitioners who are inevitably members of the communities that carry these traditions. We believe that this is the missing piece in Sloan's overall argument and that his conclusions about the relationship between medicine and religion are so strongly negative because he improperly bypasses the philosophical and theological foundations of medicine itself. Put another way, once it is conceded that reliance on normative disciplines is required in order to articulate a basic understanding of the meaning and ends of medicine, it then follows that the clinical practice of medicine is equally connected to normative understandings of the good life, the nature of humankind, and the moral and ethical aspects of the medical profession. We suggest that any who reject a relationship between medicine and spirituality have failed to adequately recognize the role that underlying norms play in their views.

Nonetheless, once we arrive at basic questions about who we really are, what is true, and the implications of our answers for curing and caring for the sick, we immediately encounter a plurality of canons and claims that find partial agreement, and irreconcilable differences. The practice of biomedicine lies at this juncture of competing moral claims and religious viewpoints. The purpose of this book is not to argue for our own particular normative claims but rather to provide anthropological snapshots, descriptions of a small but significant set of examples of the plurality of viewpoints and medical practices that are undergirded by religious or spiritual presuppositions. We do this by offering case examples of how individual physicians, operating from different spiritual traditions, practice and engage medicine in light of these traditions. There is, as ethicist Robert Veatch has suggested, no "single entity called *medicine*." Instead, "there may be as many different *medicines* as there are world views" (Veatch 2000, p. 83). Veatch's claim may exaggerate the practical differences between traditions, but the normative claims supplied by spiritual worldviews and undergirding medical practice are irreducibly plural.

While we do not necessarily see pluralism as a good in itself, we do suggest that the context of pluralism increases individual recognition of the need to exercise self-reflection—a virtuous practice in its own right. Physicians are in dire need of reflecting on their own motivations and medical practices in order to understand both themselves and the work they do. Without critical self-examination, we all risk losing our own souls and the soul of the profession. Self-examination is necessary not only for religious minorities, who are acutely aware of their presuppositions because they are markedly distinct from the dominant medical ethos. It is also important for the many physicians who have little awareness of their personal identity, motivations, or perspectives on how medicine relates to the most basic questions of life. In our framework, all physicians, religious and irreligious, spiritual and nonspiritual, need to identify the moral, philosophical, and theological traditions that locate us all, and then need to reflect upon and discuss how our own traditions shape our practice of medicine.

The Clinical Relevance Model for Spirituality and Religion

The dominant medical ethos does not take into account how philosophical and theological traditions shape medical practice. It may be another generation before the framework that we propose might be openly received and implemented. In the meantime, we suggest an incremental approach to this subject using a model which might be termed the "clinical relevance model for spirituality and religion." This is not a normative model in the sense that this is the way it should be for all time. Instead, it acknowledges that the medical profession is currently organized primarily around the physical and psychological, rather than around other dimensions of the person or patient. While the experience of illness is complex and impinges on environmental and transcendent domains (Sulmasy 2006b), the social role currently expected of physicians is to focus on physical and mental disorders. The clinical relevance model assumes that the more clearly a religious or spiritual issue is connected to the treatment of one of these physical or mental disorders, the more clearly a physician is obligated to understand and engage that issue. In these circumstances, there is a social mandate for physicians to provide some level of spiritual care. Disavowing this mandate overlooks how the physical, the emotional, and the spiritual can intertwine in the experience of illness.

In the rest of this chapter, we present this model under the headings of why, when, how, what, what next, where and who.

Why

In addition to the above philosophical foundation for envisioning an integrated relationship between spirituality and medicine, at least three lines of evidence support the involvement of clinicians in their patients' spiritual lives. The scientific literature on religion and health outcomes shows a positive correlation between measures of religiousness and health in a wide range of psychiatric and medical conditions (Koenig, McCullough, and Larson 2001). Most patients surveyed want their physicians to inquire about their spirituality (Steinhauser et al. 2000; McCord et al. 2004). And research still in its infancy points to positive medical consequences of providing spiritual care such as improved coping (Nelson et al. 2002), increased quality of life (Tarakeshwar et al. 2006; Astrow et al. 2007), less aggressive care at the end of life (Balboni et al. 2007, 2010), and lower health care costs. More study is needed to determine which elements of spirituality are best addressed in the provision of clinical care, who should provide these elements, and when and in which settings they are optimally provided.

When

When to engage spiritual concerns depends on answers to more fundamental questions: What is spirituality? What is its role in illness and health? What is health (or optimal functioning)? What is the clinician's role in the patient's life? An adequate exploration of these questions is beyond the scope of this chapter, but we believe it is important to clarify our assumptions about them.

Recognizing that spirituality continues to be difficult to define precisely, we here accept the emerging consensus that spirituality refers generally to one's relationship to a larger, or transcendent, context that gives life meaning (Puchalski et al. 2009; Koenig 2008; Sulmasy 2006a). Religion, by comparison, refers to beliefs and practices shared by a particular spiritual community. While it has become common to contrast spirituality with religion, particularly as more individualistic Westerners describe themselves as "spiritual but not religious," Wuthnow (1998) points out that the spiritual practices of the nonreligious also tend to become social, rule-guided, and dependent on tradition.

Every defining concept has limitations related to underlying presuppositions and context. For example, Harold Koenig (2008) points out the limitations of "religion" for capturing human experience, and of "spirituality" for measuring that experience. However, since most people continue to conceptualize both terms as having slightly different meanings but being normally tethered together, we prefer to retain both, referring to "religion or spirituality."

With regard to its relationship to health and illness, we follow the World Health Organization's definition of health as "a state of complete physical, mental and social well-being and not merely the absence of disease or infirmity" (WHO 1948) and agree with the draft position paper by the World Psychiatric Association's Section on Religion, Spirituality and Psychiatry, which reads in part: "Spirituality and religion are concerned with the core beliefs, values and experiences of human beings. A consideration of their relevance to the origins, understanding and treatment of psychiatric disorders should therefore be a central part of clinical and academic psychiatry. Spiritual and religious considerations also have important ethical implications for the clinical practice of psychiatry. In particular, it is affirmed here that . . . spiritual well-being, as indicated in the WHO definition of health, is an important aspect of health" (P. Verhagen, personal communication, 29 Sept. 2008). This holistic view is consistent with that articulated by Hall, Koenig, and Meador (2004) that differing religious or spiritual traditions, rather than being "frostings" on the cake of a generic, objective secular account of the human condition, each "constitute self-satisfying, cultural-linguistic worldviews" (p. 389) that provide a comprehensive interpretation of that condition without requiring reference to any external narrative or tradition. A practical implication of this is that differing worldviews need to be engaged on their own terms, much as one would learn a language.

In our view, physicians have an important role in promoting the health of the whole person and in relieving suffering, as well as in diagnosing and treating disease. We therefore agree with Curlin and Hall (2005) that the current prevailing paradigm regarding spirituality and religion overly limits the scope of the physician-patient dialogue. They characterize this approach as a form of therapeutic technique, engaged by one stranger, the physician, upon another stranger, the patient, which focuses on questions of physicians' competence, threats to patients' autonomy, and neutrality. Instead, they argue that dialogue regarding spirituality is better approached as a form of moral discourse about ultimate human concerns which is often essential to the patient-physician relationship, and one most appropriately guided by an ethic of moral friendship that seeks the patient's good through wisdom.

While morality and spirituality are always constitutive of the patient-physician relationship, consciousness of this dynamic usually remains under the surface. Under what conditions, therefore, would a clinician directly acknowledge and engage spiritual experiences, beliefs, and values in the service of seeking a patient's good as a moral friend? Evidence is accumulating about how patients experience spirituality within the medical setting (Moadel et al. 1999; Sulmasy 2006a; Alcorn et al. 2010). While one could argue that spiritual care should follow their experience, what normally most concerns the clinician is how the patient's spirituality directly impinges on the challenges of relieving distress, treating disease, and promoting recovery and health.

Spiritual distress is exemplified by the anguished question of the mother of a child with leukemia who asks, "Why did God do this to me?" Research has shown that spiritual concerns vary (Moadel et al. 1999; Astrow et al. 2007; Alcorn et al. 2010), but that they are common. For example, Alcorn and associates found that even among patients who reported that religion or spirituality was not important to their experience of illness, 67 percent reported 1–3 spiritual concerns and 40 percent reported 4 or more.

The theological convictions of some religious groups can conflict with recommended medical treatment (Koenig 2004). A familiar example is a Jehovah's Witness patient who refuses to accept a potentially life-saving blood transfusion. And patients may lack spiritual resources that could contribute to their recovery—for example, in the form of relationships with a religious or spiritual community (Peteet 1993). Consider the patient attempting to overcome addiction to marijuana who wishes he could better develop his inner life but has difficulty returning to the Catholic church because a priest abused him.

The ways that religious or spiritual beliefs, experiences, and values cause distress, interfere with treatment, or reveal clinically relevant needs, rather than defining the boundaries of the physician's role, suggest ways that spirituality is most likely to impinge on the center of the physician's task. For example, if two cancer patients believe they are being punished by God, but this belief is affecting only one of the patients' treatment decisions (such as via refusal of treatment), a clinical relevance model would suggest that spiritual care from a clinician is more appropriate in the case of one patient than the other. This does not imply that the spiritual concern experienced by the other patient is unimportant, only that it is more distant from the central focus of the clinician. Whether a physician should address spiritual needs that are not directly related to the patient's illness depends on many other factors, such as the nature of the personal relationship between the doctor and the patient, their agreement to address such concerns, the clinician's expertise, the availability of other resources, the clinician's own religious or spiritual beliefs and experiences, and the potential for interference with the clinician's primary task. (See the discussion below, under "Psychotherapeutic Sessions.")

How

A growing number of policy-making organizations, including the National Consensus Project for Quality Palliative Care, the National Comprehensive Cancer Centers Network (NCCN), and the Joint Commission recommend that spiritual assessment be part of routine clinical care. While screening tools can serve as useful memory prompts, the most natural approach is for a clinician to listen actively for what is most important to the patient, for the patient's experiences of transcendence, for specific spiritual concerns (e.g., questioning "why me?" or believing that illness is a punishment), and for problems the patient has in using religious or spiritual resources (e.g., spiritual practices, a community, or a pastor). Active listening will suggest additional, clarifying questions about the content of these domains (see below, under "What" and "What Next"). Tools intended for routine screening, such as the FICA instrument (table 2.1), can also help prompt clinicians to ask about spirituality issues with a view to their clinical relevance. Once identified, these can then be incorporated into a comprehensive formulation of the patient's case, as factors that contribute either risk or protection.

What

Many health care organizations satisfy their mandate to assess spirituality by simply asking for a patient's religious identification. While it is important to acknowledge the extent of religious diversity in the world (table 2.2), this approach is limiting, since many individuals are only nominally religious. Surveys have reported that between 9 percent (Curlin et al. 2005) and 24 percent of adults in the United States describe themselves as "spiritual but not reli-

Table 2.1. The FICA instrument

F	*Faith and belief* Do you consider yourself to be a spiritual or religious person? What is your faith or belief?	If the patient answers "yes" to the first question, the physician can continue with the other questions. If the answer is "no," the physician might ask: "What gives your life meaning?" Patients sometimes respond to this with answers such as family, nature, and careers.
I	*Importance and influence* What importance does faith have in your life? Have your beliefs influenced the way you take care of yourself and your illness? What role do your beliefs play in regaining your health?	
C	*Community* Are you a part of a spiritual or religious community? Is this of support to you and how? Is there a group of people you really love or who are important to you?	Communities such as churches, temples, synagogues, or masjids can serve as a strong support system for some patients.
A	*Address in care* How would you like me to address these issues in your health care?	

Source: Puchalski and Romer 2000.

gious" (Beliefnet 2005). Others do not think of themselves as spiritual. Assessing the relevant domains of spirituality is challenging not only because, as noted above, spirituality has been difficult to define but also because caregivers have found it difficult to agree on which of its dimensions deserve emphasis in the medical setting.

Dozens of published research instruments and suggested questions for caregivers now exist (e.g., Fitchett 2002; Hodge 2003; Atchley 2009). Some focus on the domains that spiritual expression can take. For example, the 2003 report by the Fetzer Institute and the National Institute on Aging Working Group, "Multidimensional Measurement of Religiousness/Spirituality for Use in Health Research" (Fetzer 2003) distinguished a number of areas, based on conceptual or theoretical considerations as well as on empirical evidence linking these areas to health: daily spiritual experiences, meaning, values, beliefs, private religious practices, religious or spiritual coping, religious support, and

Table 2.2. Basic information on world religions

Religion	Date founded	Sacred texts	Membership (millions)	% of world
Christianity	30 CE	Bible	2,039	32
Islam	622 CE	Qur'an, Hadith	1,226	19
Hinduism	1500 BCE (and much older roots)	Bhagavad-Gita, Upanishads, Rig Veda	828	13
No religion	—	—	775	12
Chinese folk religion	270 BCE	None	390	6
Buddhism	523 BCE	Tripitaka, Sutras	364	6
Tribal religions, Shamanism, Animism	Prehistory	Oral tradition	232	4
Atheism	—	—	150	2
New religions	Various	Various	103	2
Sikhism	1500 CE	Guru Granth Sahib	23.8	<1
Judaism	Second millennium BCE	Torah, Tanach, Talmud	14.5	<1
Spiritism	—	—	12.6	<1
Baha'i	1863 CE	Alkitab Alaqdas	7.4	<1
Confucianism	520 BCE	Lun Yu	6.3	<1
Jainism	570 BCE	Siddhanta, Pakrit	4.3	<1
Zoroastrianism	600–6000 BCE	Avesta	2.7	<1
Shinto	500 CE	Kojiki, Nohon Shoki	2.7	<1
Taoism	550 BCE	Tao-te-Ching	2.7	<1
Other	Various	Various	1.1	<1
Wicca	Ancient: 800 BCE; Modern: 1940 CE	None	No reliable measure	<1

Source: www.religioustolerance.org/worldrel.htm, accessed 5 Sept. 2009.

so on. Others emphasize the content of religious or spiritual beliefs and values (King et al. 2006). Still others, believing that subjective spiritual experience is of primary importance, focus on this dimension (Atchley 2009). And others focus on potentially beneficial outcomes—that is, on spiritual well-being (Gomez and Fisher 2003). For example, the Functional Assessment of Chronic Illness Therapy—Spiritual Well-Being Scale (FACIT-Sp) for measuring quality of life in patients who have cancer asks respondents about how much they feel a sense of purpose, peace, harmony, and meaning (Peterman et al. 2002).

While attention to each of these dimensions (domains including subjective experience, content, and outcome) can provide useful information about a patient's overall functioning, from the perspective of clinical relevance it is most helpful to ascertain how spirituality functions in the patient's experiences of illness and healing Specifically, a clinician will be listening for how his patient's spiritual values, practices, beliefs, relationships, and experiences are either helpful resources or problems (e.g., in the form of ambivalently held relationships, competing values, unavailable practices, burdensome beliefs, or painful experiences). Put another way, a clinician most needs to understand how well the patient's spirituality functions to address the core concerns of his or her life as they are activated by illness.

What Next?

Where should spiritual assessment lead? From the perspective of clinical relevance, it should inform the clinician's understanding of what impairs and what enhances the patient's functioning in the world in areas of existential concern such as identity, hope, meaning or purpose, morality, and autonomy and relationship to authority (Yalom 1980; Griffith and Griffith 2002; Griffith and Gaby 2005). This understanding, or clinical formulation, in turn serves as the basis of the clinician's use of spiritual interventions.

Identity. A person's identity, or core sense of self over time, often has a transcendent dimension that is unmasked by life events such as a serious illness. A work-oriented business executive who wonders after a heart attack if he is the same person might decide, "This experience has helped me see what I value most" or "I know I am loved or worthwhile because God loves me." Such understandings are facilitated by a spirituality that is engaged and transformative rather than static. For example, the patient might recall and identify with the Four Noble Truths of Buddhism or with the teaching of Jesus that one must lose one's life in order to save it. A clinician who appreciates that a patient is suffering from a static spirituality might appropriately explore what resources in his life had previously engaged his imagination and what obstacles exist to returning to them.

Hope. Hope is vital to coping effectively with serious illness (Groopman 2004).When a loss or a serious illness shakes a religious person's faith, he or she can become cynical or despairing. Nonreligious patients whose hopes are ultimately grounded in transcendent ideals such as compassion, truth, or justice may also be vulnerable to despair if disillusioned by the circumstances of their illness or by the behavior of individuals who have represented these ideals in their lives. As Judith Herman (1992) points out in her book *Trauma and Recovery*, a survivor of trauma needs help to reconstruct her fragmented view of the world. Clinicians who work with patients who have lost hope are familiar with the task of helping them to find a spirituality that is integrated rather than ambivalent or torn.

Meaning or purpose. Many individuals bring into treatment their search for purpose and the larger meaning of their suffering (Yalom 1980; Herman 1992). An atheist who loses a child to cancer may question whether his life has any purpose. A religious trauma survivor may question whether he can continue to believe that God is fair or loving (Peteet 2001). A depressed patient may fear that he is being punished for an unpardonable sin. Patients searching for meaning benefit from a spirituality that is contemplative and attuned rather than distracted, impulsive, or self-centered. Mindfulness and meaning-centered therapies address this need. Patients who report finding meaning may also report belief in God's will and increased companionship with God (Alcorn et al. 2010).

Morality. Patients often present with struggles that have moral aspects, including knowing what is the right thing to do, actually doing it, dealing with moral failure, or developing character (Peteet 2004). These are shaped by one's worldview in several ways. A person's understanding of God and of the universe underlies commitments to justice, caring, honesty, and community. Philosophical or religious ways of thinking (e.g., depending on, versus questioning, authority) guide the way people make moral decisions. Religious traditions articulate standards of right and wrong as well as offer options for dealing with moral failure (e.g., confession, forgiveness, making amends). Faith-based communities and community service organizations help support virtues that are basic to clinical work, such as integrity, equanimity, humility, honesty, and caring.

Regardless of differences in worldviews, patients who have moral concerns benefit from a spirituality that is mature rather than underdeveloped. Hospital chaplains are familiar with the task of helping adults who are facing a crisis to call on a conception of spirituality that goes beyond what they took from childhood (for example, in Sunday School). This task involves helping them to build on their core beliefs, which they may have not thought much about, a framework that is consonant with their chronological age and capable of addressing their present-day illness. James Fowler (1995), in his book *Stages of Faith*, describes ways in which faith development, like moral and emotional development, progresses through expectable phases. Here the clinician's task is not to suggest a more "mature" view of the world but to help the patient to draw on his own tradition in overcoming delays in his or her spiritual development.

Autonomy and relationship to authority. The worldviews of religious and nonreligious individuals differ sharply on the question of their relationship to an ultimate authority. These differences tend to emerge most clearly when dealing with distress over "unfair" pain, a decision about an unwanted pregnancy, a new realization of sexual identity, a question of withdrawal of life support, or a desire to "end it all." Is there an external authority (God, the Other, Creation) whom one can trust for support, care, and direction, or does one need to rely on oneself? Whatever one's worldview, it seems better (for the sake of this relationship, as well as for emotional reasons), to feel loved than to feel rejected by such an external authority, as Pargament's (1997) research suggests. In the story of the reunion of the Hebrew father and the prodigal son, the father lovingly accepts the return of a repentant and destitute son, who had arrogantly demanded his inheritance, left for distant lands, and squandered everything on sinful living. The father, rather than being an authority who resented his son's autonomy, was more ready to receive the lost son than the son could imagine. It can sometimes be important for the therapeutic plan for a patient who blames his illness on bad choices to recognize that love, forgiveness, and intimacy are still possible.

A comprehensive diagnostic formulation identifies whether a need exists to address spiritual distress and then resources (or obstacles) that a patient's spirituality presents to achieving the goals of care. This involves determining whether the patient's spirituality is helpful or unhelpful in dealing with his or her core concerns (i.e., whether that spirituality is engaged versus static, integrated versus torn or ambivalent, contemplative versus distracted, mature versus developmentally delayed, based on love versus rejection). Consider the following examples: a woman with a previously engaged relationship with God whose major depression is complicated by distress over loss of faith and who now feels unable to pray; anxiety in a man facing surgery who is feeling guilty for his prior mistreatment of his children and is disconnected from his church; and an athlete disabled by an injury who is coping with a loss of meaning and would like to return to meditation.

Where

In many modern clinical settings, speed and complaint-specific focused diagnosis and treatment are the expectation. A comprehensive clinical formulation, even without a spiritual component, is rare and often impractical to achieve. A clinician's approach will therefore vary according to the setting. Examples to consider are focused contacts for urgent care; office visits for nonurgent problems; psychotherapeutic sessions; care in religiously affiliated health care institutions; and discussions near the end of life.

Focused Contacts for Urgent Care

A patient presenting to an emergency room in distress, or to an anesthesiologist with extreme anxiety and second thoughts about major surgery, requires rapid assessment. Asking what is bothering or worrying the patient most may uncover fears about losing control, being alone, or being unable to care for others. Knowing the patient's usual supports can help the clinician connect the patient with resources, including spiritual ones he or she has used before. For example, in the preoperative holding area, a cardiac patient tells the anesthesiologist that last night he and his wife opened and enjoyed a bottle of wine they had been saving for 30 years. What might the patient be trying to communicate to the physician, and does it make any difference to the clinical plan? One could gloss over the remark because the immediate need is to finish the history and physical exam before the upcoming interventional coronary revascularization in the catheterization lab. Or one could take it as an invitation to delve further and ask why the patient and his wife opened that bottle of wine. The answer—an overwhelming fear of certain death—could predict the high possibility of extreme resistance to sedative-hypnotics during surgery, with a subsequent fatal loss of airway because of inadvertent oversedation. A physician needs to be comfortable asking a question that could be spiritually charged. In this case, the patient's answer to such a question prompted a potentially life-saving change of plan from sedation to general anesthesia using a protected airway.

Office Visits for Nonurgent Care

Patients want their primary care physicians to know who they are as people. Perhaps for this reason, studies indicate that a majority of outpatients want their physicians to ask about their religious or spiritual lives (McCord et al. 2004). While spiritual issues rarely come up explicitly in nonurgent office visits, most patients want their physicians to be able to help them make important decisions when serious illness strikes. Openness to hearing about what matters most to the patients, and why, also establishes a basis for trust. Some patients want to be able to ask questions that may be more explicitly spiritual, such as "Why is this happening to me?" The clinician may then decide to address such questions in a psychotherapeutic context, or refer them to an appropriate spiritual resource, such as a chaplain.

Psychotherapeutic Sessions

Over the past 20 years, interest has grown in integrating spirituality into psychotherapy (Griffith and Griffith 2002; Josephson and Peteet 2004; Sperry and Shafranske 2005; Pargament 2007). While a review of this literature is beyond the scope of this chapter, a few considerations deserve mention here.

One is the availability of four different approaches to spiritual problems (Peteet 1994). In the most familiar and straightforward of these, a therapist would acknowledge the problem but limit discussion to its psychological dimension. For example, she might address a patient's anger with God by examining his relationship with other authority figures.

A second approach would be to clarify the worldview as well as the psychological aspects of the problem, suggest resources for dealing with the former, and consider working with an outside resource such as a religious community or other authority. This might include enlisting a hospital chaplain or clergyperson to offer spiritual help or referring a patient to a therapist of a similar tradition or worldview. It might also include referral to a program that integrates beliefs and emotions, such as a religiously or spiritually based cognitive behavioral program (Probst et al. 1992; Bilu and Witztum 1993) or a twelve-step program.

In a third approach, the clinician would aim to address the problem indirectly using the patient's own philosophy of life. This might include exploring ways the patient can make better use of his or her resources and tradition (e.g., by examining a range of beliefs in the patient's own denomination or correcting misconceptions about the spiritual foundation of Alcoholics Anonymous).

A fourth approach would be to address the problem directly together using a shared perspective in the case that physician and patient share a common worldview. This approach could range from the therapist's agreement on the importance of hope, meaning, worldview, or a caring community to the prescriptive use of shared values, beliefs, or practices (e.g., meditation or scripture) in the treatment. Careful attention to transference, countertransference, boundary, and consent issues is critical here. Of course, there may be times when clinicians need to engage directly the value dimension of spiritual problems without the benefit of a shared world view. Referring to shared values and to the patient's moral functioning can serve as a guide (Peteet 2004).

To choose among these approaches, a clinician needs to keep in mind several additional considerations. One is the usefulness of identifying and prioritizing goals, which then imply different therapeutic strategies. Is the primary goal in a given case to treat a recognized disorder, to relieve suffering, or to improve functioning? For example, if the patient's spiritual problem is interfering with effective treatment of an emotional condition, an appropriate strategy might be to address it until it is no longer interfering. If spiritual distress is clinically significant, the strategy might be to relieve it by helping the patient resolve the concern. And if a spiritual need is impeding progress toward optimal functioning, the strategy could be to help the patient find a way to meet that need.

Tactics follow from these strategies. Religiously based cognitive behavioral therapy for depression is an example of a way to help a patient resolve religiously reinforced distortions of perspective (Probst et al. 1992). Tactics for addressing unmet spiritual needs include identifying what resources have sustained the patient in the past and what the patient's relationship now is to them. For example, what spiritual practices (e.g., meditation, listening to music, communing with nature, or praying) has the patient found helpful? Galanter et al. (2009) has reviewed ways of incorporating spirituality as a resource within a group format for psychiatric or primary care patients who have HIV/AIDS, cancer, or addictive disorders.

It is also important to consider the transference, countertransference, and ethical implications of dealing with patients' spirituality. Patients often develop strong unconscious responses to clinicians based on their perception of the clinician's worldview. For example, patients who believe (or suspect, for example, on the basis of the clinician's name) that their clinician shares their worldview may unconsciously respond based on formative experiences with religious authority figures. Patients are often more likely to trust a physician who understands and shares important values and beliefs. On the other hand, they may be ashamed to share their moral failings with a clinician of the same faith. A patient who knows or assumes that a clinician has a different worldview can suspect the clinician of undermining cherished values or may also regard the clinician as safer and more objective than someone from the patient's own tradition. Physicians can also respond unconsciously to patients depending on whether they share the same worldview. In the same tradition, a clinician may respond to a patient's conservatism by reacting as he did to his fundamentalist father's, or may attempt to enlighten a younger patient with whom he identifies. A physician of a patient from a different tradition may recoil from religious beliefs she finds personally repugnant.

These unconscious responses of patients and physicians may interact in ways that become complementary (e.g., parent-child or seeker-teacher), encourage merging (as when a sense of religious intimacy leads to avoidance of needed confrontation), stimulate oppositional struggles (with engagement of old conflicts with religious authority), or develop in even more complex ways (Abernathy and Lancia 1998).

Finally, boundary considerations apply, such as how to deal with patients' questions about the therapist's own spiritual identification. We consider these in the chapter devoted to ethical issues and professionalism (chapter 12).

Religiously Affiliated Institutions

Health care institutions that have clear ties to religious organizations or communities create a unique context in which spiritual care may be delivered. Over 15 percent of hospitals in the United States alone are composed of institutions governed by the Roman Catholic Church. There also remain many other smaller doctors' offices and clinics that have clear religious missions. In the developing world many mission hospitals have religious goals tethered to the provision of medical care. Spiritual care in such institutional contexts takes a variety of forms based on the beliefs and practices of the governing religious communities, but practitioners often feel freer in these than in other settings to include spiritual along with clinical guidance, scripture readings, and prayer.

Discussions near the End of Life

The prospect of dying puts into stark relief questions about identity, hope, meaning or purpose, guilt, and one's relationship to ultimate authority. Recognizing this, the specialty of palliative medicine has as one of its goals the relief of spiritual distress, and Sulmasy (2006a, b) has described ways of incorporating spiritual into end of life care. Narrative approaches (Viederman and Perry 1980) as well as meaning-centered approaches (Breitbart and Heller 2003) have demonstrated usefulness here. The following case illustrates the way in which a medical team distinguished between treatment and healing to approach a patient's religious objection to accepting treatment for cancer.

A woman hospitalized for recently diagnosed cancer emphasized that she was looking to God to cure her illness. Her medical team feared that she would refuse recommended treatment as being inconsistent with her faith, and they discussed with clinicians who had known her longer how best to approach her. Subsequently, her oncologist approached her by saying that the team recognized her strong faith, that many of the hospital staff were also believers, that their role was to offer treatments, and that only God could heal. She agreed to accept the team's recommendations.

At times, collaboration with the patient's spiritual authority can be crucial. A mother of two in her forties who had metastatic cervical cancer refused opiates for pain because of her belief in healing through Christian Science. As she approached death, her family and the hospital staff caring for her became increasingly distressed at witnessing her suffering. Eventually, they conferred with the patient's Christian Science practitioner, who helped her see that the choice of how much to rely on medication was her own to make and not one prescribed by her religion.

Who

Because of physicians' limited time, comfort, and expertise in dealing with spiritual issues, some argue that clinicians should screen and that chaplains should assess and intervene (Puchalski and Romer 2009). While fully endorsing the multidisciplinary model of care and recognizing the practical constraints on physicians' practices, we believe that many physicians can provide spiritual care, and that many chaplains can serve as consultants as well as spiritual providers, helping to teach their clinical colleagues how to respond to their shared patients' spiritual concerns.

As we suggested at the outset of this chapter, self-awareness is essential to effectively responding to spiritual concerns. More specifically: How aware are potential providers of the values undergirding their practice? How aware are they of where they fit personally within the philosophical or religious tradition of which they are a part? How integrated is their spirituality with their own practice, and how aware are they of tensions at this interface? How do they deal with the culture of biomedicine and with patients who hold different religious or spiritual beliefs? How experienced are they with the opportunities and potential pitfalls of engaging the spiritual lives of their patients? How well do they nurture their own spiritual lives? Subsequent chapters provide examples of how physicians within differing traditions address these questions.

Conclusion

This brief chapter emphasizes, and those that follow illustrate, that each clinician needs to understand his own orientation to life and healing and to develop an approach to dealing with the spiritual dimension of life and death which is consistent with the nature of his or her particular practice. Appreciating the importance of spiritual concerns to individuals made vulnerable by illness can lead to more active listening for these concerns, to connecting more effectively with patients about what matters most to them (Atchley 2009), and, where indicated by the clinical situation, to enhancing their functioning by assisting them with these concerns. Mastering these skills enables the physician to enhance both the therapeutic interaction and the patient's healing.

REFERENCES

Abernathy, J. D., and J. J. Lancia. 1998. Religion and the psychotherapeutic relationship: Transferential and countertransferential dimensions. *Journal of Psychotherapy Practice and Research* 7:281–89.

Alcorn, S. A., M. J. Balboni, H. G. Prigerson, A. Reynolds, A. C. Phelps, A. A. Wright, S. D. Block, J. R. Peteet, L. A. Kachnic, and T. A. Balboni. 2010. "If God wanted me yesterday, I wouldn't be here today": Religious and spiritual themes in patients' experiences of advanced cancer. *Journal of Palliative Medicine* 13:581–88.

Astrow, A. B., A. Wexler, K. Texeira, M. Ki He, and D. P. Sulmasy. 2007. Is failure to meet spiritual needs associated with cancer patients' perceptions of quality of care and their satisfaction with care? *Journal of Clinical Oncology* 25:5753–57.

Atchley, R. C. 2009. *Spirituality and Aging*. Baltimore, MD: Johns Hopkins University Press.

Balboni, T. A., T. A. Vanderwerker, S. D. Block, M. E. Paulk, C. S. Lathan, J. R. Peteet, and H. J. Prigerson. 2007. Religiousness and spiritual support among advanced cancer patients and associations with end-of-life treatment preferences and quality of life. *Journal of Clinical Oncology* 25:467–68.

Balboni, T. A., M. E. Paulk, M. J. Balboni, A. C. Phelps, E. T. Loggers, A. A. Wright, S. D. Block, E. F. Lewis, J. R. Peteet, and H. G. Prigerson. 2010. Provision of spiritual care to patients with advanced cancer: Associations with medical care and quality of life near death. *Journal of Clinical Oncology* 28:445–52.

Beliefnet. 2005. Newsweek / Beliefnet poll results. www.beliefnet.com/News/2005/08/Newsweekbeliefnet-Poll-Results.aspx#spiritrel. Accessed 19 June 2010.

Bilu, Y., and E. Witztum. 1993. Working with Jewish Ultra-Orthodox patients: Guidelines for culturally sensitive therapy. *Culture, Medicine and Psychiatry* 17:197–233.

Breitbart, W., and K. S. Heller. 2003. Reframing hope: Meaning-centered care for patients near the end of life. *Journal of Palliative Medicine* 6:979–88.

Curlin, F. A., and D. E. Hall. 2005. Strangers or friends: A proposal for a new spirituality-in-medicine ethic. *Journal of General Internal Medicine* 20:370–74.

Curlin, F. A., J. D. Lantos, C. J. Roach, S. A. Sellergren, and M. H. Chin. 2005. Religious characteristics of U.S. physicians: A national survey. *Journal of General Internal Medicine* 20:629–34.

Fetzer Institute. 2003. *Multidimensional Measurement of Religiousness/Spirituality for Use in Health Research.* A report of the Fetzer Institute and the National Institute on Aging Working Group. Kalamazoo, MI.

Fitchett, G. 2002. *Assessing Spiritual Needs: A Guide for Caregivers.* Lima, OH: Academic Renewal Press.

Fowler, J. W. 1995. *Stages of Faith: The Psychology of Faith and the Quest for Meaning.* New York: HarperCollins.

Galanter, M. 2009. The concept of spirituality in relation to addiction recovery and general psychiatry. In *Recent Developments in Alcoholism*, pp. 1–16. New York: Springer.

Gomez, R., and J. W. Fisher. 2003. Domains of spiritual well-being and development and validation of the Spiritual Well-Being Questionnaire. *Personality and Individual Differences* 35:1975–91.

Griffith, J. L., and L. Gaby. 2005. Brief psychotherapy at the bedside: Countering demoralization from medical illness. *Psychosomatics* 46:109–16.

Griffith, J. L., and M. E. Griffith. 2002. *Encountering the Sacred: How to Talk with People about Their Spiritual Lives.* New York: Guilford Press.

Groopman, J. 2004. *The Anatomy of Hope.* New York. Random House.

Hall, D. E., H. G. Koenig, and K. G. Meador. 2004. Conceptualizing religion: How language shapes and constrains knowledge in the study of religion and health. *Perspectives in Biology and Medicine* 47:386–401.

Herman, J. 1992. *Trauma and Recovery: The Aftermath of Violence—From Domestic Violence to Political Terror.* New York: Basic Books.

Hodge, D. R. 2003. *Spiritual Assessment: Handbook for Helping Professionals.* Botford, CT: National Association of Christians in Social Work.

Josephson, A. J., and J. R. Peteet, eds. 2004. *Handbook of Spirituality and Worldview in Clinical Practice.* Washington, DC: American Psychiatric Publishing.

King, M., L. Jones, K. Barnes, J. Low, C. Walker, S. Wilkinson, C. Mason, J. Sutherland, and A. Tookman. 2006. Measuring spiritual belief: Development and standardization of a beliefs and values scale. *Psychological Medicine* 36:417–25.

Koenig, H. G. 2004. Religion, spirituality, and medicine: Research findings and implications for clinical practice. *Southern Medical Journal* 97:1194–1200.

———. 2008. *Medicine, Religion and Health: Where Science and Spirituality Meet.* West Conshocken, PA: Templeton Foundation Press.

Koenig, H. G., M. E. McCullough, and D. B. Larson. 2001. *Handbook of Religion and Health.* New York: Oxford University Press.

MacIntyre, A. C. 1984. *After Virtue: A Study in Moral Theory.* 2nd ed. Notre Dame, IN: University of Notre Dame Press.

McCord, G., V. J. Gilchrist, S. D. Grossman, B. D. King, K. F. McCormick, A. M. Oprandi, S. L. Schrop, et al. 2004. Discussing spirituality with patients: A rational and ethical approach. *Annals of Family Medicine* 2:356–61.

Moadel, A., C. Morgan, A. Fatone, J. Grennan, J. Carter, G. Laruffa, A. Skummy, and J. Dutcher. 1999. Seeking meaning and hope: Self-reported spiritual and existential needs among an ethnically-diverse cancer patient population. *Psycho-Oncology* 8:378–85.

Nelson, C. J., B. J. Rosenfeld, W. Breitbart, and M. Galietta. 2002. Spirituality, religion and depression in the terminally ill. *Psychosomatics* 43:213–20.

Pargament, K. I. 1997. *The Psychology of Religion and Coping: Theory, Research, Practice.* New York: Guilford Press.

———. 2007. *Spiritually Integrated Psychotherapy: Understanding and Addressing the Sacred.* New York: Guilford Press.

Peteet, J. R. 1993. A closer look at the role of a spiritual approach in addictions treatment. *Journal of Substance Abuse Treatment* 10:263–67.

———. 1994. Approaching religious issues in psychotherapy: A conceptual framework. *Journal of Psychotherapy Practice and Research* 3:237–45.

———. 2001. Putting suffering into perspective: Implications of the patient's world view. *Journal of Psychotherapy Practice and Research* 10:187–92.

———. 2004. *Doing the Right Thing: An Approach to Moral Issues in Mental Health Treatment.* Washington, DC: American Psychiatric Publishing.

Peterman, A. H., G. Fitchett, M. J. Brady, L. Hernandez, and D. Cella. 2002. Measuring spiritual well-being in people with cancer: The functional assessment of chronic illness therapy—Spiritual Well-being Scale (FACIT- Sp). *Annals of Behavioral Medicine* 24:49–58.

Probst, L. R., R. Ostrom, P. Watkins, T. Dean, and D. Mashburn. 1992. Comparative efficacy of religious and nonreligious cognitive-behavioral therapy for the treatment of clinical depression in religious individuals. *Journal of Consulting and Clinical Psychology* 60:94–103.

Puchalski, C., B. Ferrell, R. Virani, S. Otis-Green, P. Baird, J. Bull, H. Chochinov, et al. 2009. Improving the quality of spiritual care as a dimension of palliative care: The report of the Consensus Conference. *Journal of Palliative Medicine* 10:885–904.

Puchalski, C., and A. L. Romer. 2000. Taking a spiritual history allows clinicians to understand patients more fully. *Journal of Palliative Medicine* 3:129–37.

Shuman, J. J., and K. G. Meador. 2003. *Heal Thyself: Spirituality, Medicine and the Distortion of Christianity.* New York: Oxford University Press.

Sloan, R. P. 2006. *Blind Faith: The Unholy Alliance of Religion and Medicine.* New York: St. Martin's.

Sperry, L., and E. P. Shafranske. 2005. *Spiritually Oriented Psychotherapy.* Washington, DC: American Psychological Association.

Steinhauser, K. E., N. A. Christakis, E. C. Clipp, M. McNeilly, L. McIntyre, and J. A. Tulsky. 2000. Factors considered important at the end of life by patients, family, physicians, and other care providers. *JAMA* 284:2476–82.

Sulmasy, D. P. 2006a. Spiritual issues in the care of the dying . . . "It's OK between me and God." *JAMA* 296:1385–92.

———. 2006b. *The Rebirth of the Clinic: An Introduction to Spirituality in Health Care.* Washington, DC: Georgetown University Press.

Tarakeshwar, N., L. C. Vanderwerker, E. Paulk, M. J. Pearce, S. V. Kasl, and H. G. Prigerson. 2006. Religious coping is associated with the quality of life of patients with advanced cancer. *Journal of Palliative Medicine* 9:646–57.

Veatch, R. M. 2000. Internal and External Sources of Morality for Medicine. In *The Health Care Professional as Friend and Healer: Building on the Work of Edmund D. Pellegrino*, ed. E. D. Pellegrino, D. C. Thomasma, and J. L. Kissell, pp. 75–86. Washington, DC: Georgetown University Press.

Viederman, M., and S. Perry. 1980. Use of a psychodynamic life narrative in the treatment of depression in the physically ill. *General Hospital Psychiatry* 3:177–85.

WHO (World Health Organization). 1948. Preamble to the Constitution of the World Health Organization as adopted by the International Health Conference, New York, 19–22 June, 1946; signed on 22 July 1946 by the representatives of 61 States (Official Records of the World Health Organization, no. 2, p. 100) and entered into force on 7 April 1948.

Wuthnow, R. 1998. *After Heaven: Spirituality in America since the 1950s*. Berkeley and Los Angeles, CA: University of California Press.

Yalom, I. D. 1980. *Existential Psychotherapy*. New York: Basic Books.

PART II / Major Traditions and Medicine

CHAPTER THREE

Judaism

Steven C. Schachter, M.D., and Terry R. Bard, D.D.

Oath-taking enjoys a long and rich history in human culture. In ancient times, oaths were among the most serious commitments people could make to each other. In ancient Hebrew culture, oaths between Abraham and his slave (Genesis 24:9) and between Joseph and his father, Jacob (Genesis 47:9), exemplify verbal oaths undertaken with physical expressions that underscored their seriousness.

Oaths therefore represented a responsibility that one individual had to another. As roles in society evolved, oath-taking by an individual who assumed responsibility for many others became common. The formalization of professions in Greek times led to the creation of professional oaths of responsibility. The Hippocratic Oath for physicians in the fourth century BCE became a model for the declaration of responsibility that physicians "swear" to their fellow physicians and, by extension, to their patients.

In Jewish culture, the oldest formal precedent of any oath of responsibility for physicians dates to the sixth century CE and is attributed to Asaph ben Berakhyahu and Yohanan ben Zabda (Sefer ha-R'fuot, or *The Book of Medicines*). Another physician's oath—Daily Prayer of a Physician, or the Prayer of Maimonides—is identified with Moses Maimonides (Moshe ben Maimon;

1135–1204), an eminent rabbi, physician, and philosopher of the Middle Ages who wrote extensively on Jewish law and ethics as well as on numerous medical topics.

The Prayer of Maimonides may have actually been written by Marcus Herz (1783), a German physician and pupil of the philosopher Immanuel Kant. It first appeared in print in the late 18th century and was introduced into the medical literature in 1917 by Harry Friedenwald (see the appendix to this chapter). Irrespective of authorship, the Prayer of Maimonides has inspired generations of physicians in their practice of medicine.

In this chapter, we—as a Jewish physician (SCS) and a rabbi and medical ethicist (TRB) who have provided medical and pastoral care, respectively, for many years at a hospital founded with Jewish roots—use the Prayer of Maimonides to frame our personal perspectives on key themes in Jewish medical ethics as they apply to the clinical practice of medicine and the conduct of clinical research. Consequently, this chapter is neither a comprehensive treatment of Jewish medical ethics nor necessarily representative of the views generally held by other Jewish physicians, rabbis, and medical ethicists. These views have all been shaped, of course, by centuries of both mystical experience and rabbinical teaching.

Insights about Life and Healing

> Thou hast chosen me to watch over the life and health of Thy creatures.

The concept that Jews are a special people, with certain privileges and responsibilities, is a fundamental tenet of Jewish theology. Although the nature of this claim to uniqueness has been understood variously throughout Jewish history and among branches of Judaism, this concept of specialness is common to all and is considered to convey special responsibilities on all Jews to make the world better, *l'tikun olam* (literally, "restore the world"). In this context, physicians in Jewish culture assume special societal roles and responsibilities. Because the practice of medicine has a theological mandate, serving as a physician is regarded as both a calling and a privilege, perhaps second in prestige only to the rabbinate. Throughout the millennia, Jewish tradition has understood the physician as "God's right hand" (c. second century BCE, Sefer Ben Sira [the book of Ben Sira]) because of the physician's responsibilities for the care and preservation of human life. Just as physicians were required to do all in their power to preserve human life, individuals were required to assume their responsibility to keep out of harm's way. Jewish law therefore prohibited people from living in towns lacking a physician (Babylonian Talmud, Baba Kama 46a).

In the last two centuries, Jewish communities in the United States, beginning with energetic nickel-and-dime fundraising and eventually evolving into equally robust individual and community commitment, have generated substantial financial resources to support the establishment of hospitals with Jewish identities, especially to provide care for Jewish patients along with others and to provide places for Jewish doctors to train. Beth Israel Hospital in Boston, established by the Boston Jewish community in 1916, Michael Reese Hospital in Chicago, Mt. Sinai Hospital in New York and Cleveland, and Cedars Sinai Medical Center in Los Angeles are all examples of this early effort. Likewise, Jewish communities have supported charities that provide medical care, such as Hadassah, the Women's Zionist Organization of America.

A DOCTOR'S STORY: Steven C. Schachter

In keeping with this tradition, I was raised in a post–World War II midwestern American Jewish community that emphasized the stature of physicians in Jewish society. I was a first-born son and was expected by my family—especially my grandparents and great-grandparents, with reinforcement from the Jewish community that surrounded me —to fulfill their desire for me to become a doctor. I accepted this vision of my future without question from an early age and indeed anticipated a career in medicine with excitement, recognizing that I was fortunate to be given the resources to make this dream a reality. The expectations of my family and the Jewish community seemed infused with and inseparable from our Jewish identities and cultural values. For my family and the generations who came before, a physician simultaneously embodied several important attributes and Jewish ideals: extensive education (which no authority could ever take away, unlike property or money), social prominence and responsibility, and perhaps most important, the capacity to heal the sick. The primacy of the physician in healing those in need was inextricably connected to timeless Jewish concepts of the role of God in granting life and good health, as reflected in the Prayer of Maimonides: "Thou hast chosen me to watch over the life and health of Thy creatures."

My familial and community inculcation steered me, indeed fated me, to become a physician, and as I grew in experience and wisdom, my professional activities and Jewish values became indistinguishable, thereby continuing an unbroken Jewish tradition linking Jewish values with the pursuit and practice of medicine.

In recent years, almost all of the hospitals established by Jewish communities in the urban United States have lost their specific Jewish identities through mergers, expansions, purchases, closures, and population migrations. Many Jews and Jewish physicians remain concerned about this shift. In part, their concern is due to their manifest and hidden loyalties to what they erected and have supported. More important, they are concerned that the Jewish values they projected onto these institutions are evaporating. However, the essential value of providing health care for all, *tikun olam*, remains, assuaging some of these often-voiced laments.

Although Jews came to the United States in the earliest days of the country's formation, the largest percentage of Jewish immigrants arrived within a three-decade span, the 1880s through 1910. The first group came from Germany and the second from Eastern Europe, about 20 years later. (A third major wave of Jews emigrated to the United States from the then Soviet Union in the 1970s and 1980s.)

These groups of Jewish immigrants differed considerably from one another but were united in their concern for issues such as health care. Meanwhile, in U.S. society at large, the traditional value of study and education, particularly of sacred texts, laws, and literature, was becoming secularized. This focus on secular education and the ability to achieve control over one's destiny by secular learning began to replace the previous emphasis on religious learning. In this context, the long-standing emphasis on the physician's special role in the community provided a goal for many of the new immigrants and their children. However, poverty and the quota systems that were then in place thwarted the efforts of many Jews to gain entrance into U.S. medical schools. In spite of these barriers, a much higher percentage of Jews per capita ultimately became physicians, even though they were not always provided admitting privileges in urban hospitals. This reality contributed to the formation of the generation of clinics and hospitals founded to provide care for Jewish communities as well as for the general population.

Thus, the historical high regard for the physician in Judaism and the socioeconomic realities of early 20th-century United States both became catalysts for many young Jews to become doctors, a trend that remained important through the first seven decades of that century. Today, the number of Jews seeking admission to medical schools, although still disproportionately high (2.2% of the general population), is somewhat less than in previous decades.

How Beliefs Influence Practice

Thou hast created the human body with infinite wisdom.
Inspire me with love for my art and for Thy creatures.

Respect for the individuality of patients and for their participation in their own health care–related decisions is widely accepted and a fundamental principle in the practice of medicine today. Respect provides the basis for the interactions between physicians and patients in the context of clinical practice, clinical research, and the training of young doctors. The Prayer of Maimonides expresses these principles by stating that patients have "infinite wisdom" and that they represent God's "creatures."

Consistent with these ideas, my approach (SCS) to caring for a patient is to first establish a therapeutic partnership by listening to his or her symptoms, carefully explaining what I think is wrong in terms that are understandable to the patient, and discussing the potential next steps and solutions as best as I can. Over time, I work closely with the patient to pursue a diagnostic and treatment plan that he or she accepts and supports, one that is consistent with his or her understanding, level of commitment, and wishes. In this way, I individualize the medical care for each patient, even though symptoms or test results may be similar from one patient to the next. To me, patients are individual, unique persons who are suffering, not merely interesting cases or examples of specific diseases.

The Prayer of Maimonides also suggests that the approach to caring for patients should incorporate respect for their dignity and humanity, rather than be based on materialistic, political, or behavioral considerations: "Preserve the strength of my body and of my soul that they ever be ready to cheerfully help and support rich and poor, good and bad, enemy as well as friend. In the sufferer let me see only the human being."

The respect for patients that follows from acknowledging their autonomy is also central to the regulations that govern patient-oriented research, as formalized in the informed consent process. In part, the affirmation that persons volunteering for clinical research have autonomy derives from atrocities performed on prisoners of war and concentration camp inmates, many of them Jewish, at the hands of Nazi doctors during World War II in the name of medical research. In 1946, judges in Nuremburg, Germany, found a number of these Nazi doctors guilty of conducting cruel and lethal experimentation. Even given this history of incomprehensible torture, the judges concluded, remarkably, that human experimentation was necessary for the advancement of medical knowledge, but only when persons gave their voluntary consent, among other requirements.

In 1964, the 18th World Medical Assembly affirmed the requirement of informed consent in human experimentation in its Declaration of Helsinki, and the National Research Act of the U.S. Congress (1974) led to a document called the Belmont Report, which formed the basis of new federal regulations governing clinical research in the United States. Two of the basic principles of medical research identified by the Belmont Report were autonomy and beneficence, both of which stem from respect for patients. Autonomy describes respect for an individual's decision regarding participation in a clinical trial. To respect autonomy, investigators must present prospective subjects complete information pertaining to a study, thereby enabling them to make an informed decision about participation. Beneficence refers to the concept of always doing good, or of doing no harm. To accomplish beneficence, investigators must balance risks to the subjects of participating in the research against potential benefits to them.

A third principle of the Belmont Report—justice—emphasizes equal access to health care as well as the benefits and obligations of clinical research and is consistent with Jewish values. Coupled with the Talmudic understanding that life is a sacred gift to all living things, such that Jewish regulations with few exceptions are to be set aside to save a life, Jewish traditions provide a value template for providing thorough health care for all patients as well as for pursuing research that promotes well-being and healthy lives. These values continue to influence Jewish perspectives about the nature of health care, its provision, and its effectiveness. The modern realities of providing personalized health care to all, pursuing the finest research that supports such care, and training young physicians to achieve these goals present significant challenges for many Jews and Jewish physicians. The commoditization of health care and the transformation of the physician into a supplier and the patient into a consumer are contrary to thousands of years of Jewish thinking and values. The traditional Jewish values and roles accorded to physicians are in jeopardy of becoming extinct, and many Jewish physicians are currently wrestling with how to recast their roles to meet today's shifting expectations and realities while preserving the deeply rooted values they hold dear.

Relationship to Contemporary Medical Practice: Addressing and Accessing Spirituality in Practice

> Enable Thy creatures to alleviate their sufferings and to heal their illnesses.

While there are many admirable pursuits in the medical arts, the most important function of a physician in the minds of patients and as articulated in the Prayer of Maimonides is to alleviate substantially, if not completely, human suffering, whether physical or emotional, using any and all available tools: "Thou hast blessed Thine earth, Thy rivers and Thy mountains with healing substances; they enable Thy creatures to alleviate their sufferings and to heal their illnesses." Indeed, Jewish values suggest that medical care should extend beyond curing or mitigating the symptoms of disease to improving the quality of life of patients and to preventing disease: "Thou hast chosen me to watch over the life and health of Thy creatures."

In keeping with this concept, I (SCS) try to offer my patients any possible therapy in the hope that they will feel and function better, even in the face of an incurable disease. Suffering can be reduced through a variety of approaches, including medical treatments, compassion, or even humor. Providing compassionate care can be time-consuming, which is challenging under the usual time constraints of a typical medical practice.

Jewish tradition understands that disease prevention is life promotion. Biblical and Talmudic regulations relating to purity rites and health care provide sacred rituals in addition to health-enhancing behaviors. Ancient requirements to bathe regularly or to prepare foods and ointments carefully likely emerged from spiritual, sometimes superstitious origins; nonetheless, they frequently served to promote good health and prolong life. Human suffering was initially understood as a theological reality. Regardless of this perspective, the role of the early priests, and then of rabbis who became physicians, in reducing or removing human suffering remains a consistent theme from ancient times to the present. Increasingly, the complexity of contemporary society challenges the reduction of human suffering and the prevention of disease. Economic and social realities, poverty, and supersized meals trump most medical efforts to contain these influences. Realities such as these vex caring physicians and are in tension with the values implied in Maimonides' prayer.

The application of these values translates variously in the Jewish community. Observant Jewish physicians in all branches of Judaism sometimes experience conflicts resulting from their adherence to *halakhic* (Jewish legal) requirements and the expectations imposed by professional practice. Jewish law has wrestled with these challenges for hundreds of years. For example, observance of the Sabbath is a basic expectation and practice for most observant Jews. Biblically, work (*m'lacha*) is prohibited on the Sabbath (Deuteronomy 5; Exodus 20). In ensuing centuries, the understanding of "work" grew. Carrying objects, igniting fire (electricity), writing, and driving or riding in an automobile represent but a few of these prohibitions. However, recognizing the physician's particular role as a divine agent, particularly in matters of life and death, Jewish law has developed special accommodations for the physician who, in an emergency, may have to violate some of these strictures. In each instance, the accommodation is made in a graduated sense with the goal of reminding the physician of two obligations: caring for the sick and fulfilling Jewish law. One example for such observant physicians relates to the necessity of writing a medical note for a patient on the Sabbath. Initially, the observant physician should determine if someone else might write the note. If this is not possible, the physician may write the note with a nondominant hand. If this is not possible, the physician is to write the note by holding the pen differently from normally. These accommodations are made to perform the physician's divine responsibility to preserve life while, at the same time, keeping foremost the coexisting obligation to observe the Sabbath.

Such accommodations can become problematic for observant physicians when faced with such issues as getting to a hospital, pushing the button on an elevator, and activating electronic equipment. Some medical centers have made accommodation for these potential problems—for example, Sabbath elevators preprogrammed to stop at every floor from the beginning of the Sabbath before sundown on Friday night and ending shortly after sundown on Saturday night. In fact, some hospitals have expanded these times by one day earlier to accommodate Muslim physicians who face similar conflicts.

Observant Jewish and Muslim physicians and patients have sometimes found that religious responsibilities can be problematic in other areas as well. Dietary requirements that differ from societal norms are a primary example. Prescriptive dietary rules in both traditions take their points of departure from the concept of *kashrut* (literally "fit for use"). This concept refers to all aspects of life, including the kind of clothing one wears, the composition of both the pen (quill) and the ink used for legal documents, and what one eats. While hospitals are federally required to accommodate patients' dietary needs, no such regulation applies to the faculties and staffs. Similarly, when observant physicians take time away from their practices to observe religious holidays, they may find that they are assigned more than their share of on-call time to make up for the time. Such problems and inequities are slowly diminishing through various models of equitable accommodation. Nonetheless, they continue to persist. Current efforts toward ensuring that cultural competency exists in all U.S. health care institutions is one way by which potentially competing values can be accommodated in order to create clinical climates that reduce or eliminate such value and practice challenges for physicians, health care workers, and patients.

Continual learning and education are highly valued in Jewish tradition, particularly with regard to the study of religious doctrines. Early rabbinic literature states that the study of Torah (literally, the five books that Jewish tradition attributes to Moses) is at the pinnacle of all other contexts in Jewish culture: *Talmud torah k'neged kulam* (Torah study is equivalent to all obligations which have no boundaries [Mishnah Peah 1:1]). The traditional understanding of this statement does not restrict learning to biblical studies, however. Instead, it expands this concept to study of all Jewish texts and eventually to knowledge in general. Thus, we can understand Rabbi Gamliel's statement, echoed by others: *Talmud torah im derekh eretz*—study is to be accompanied by a worldly occupation (Pirqe Avot 2:2), which adds two dimensions to the first value. Practically, tending to one's livelihood is a tandem responsibility along with continual learning, and some might add continual questioning to the mix. From this perspective, the teacher is elevated to a special role, epitomizing learning as well as becoming a practical role model for others. Thus, *rabbi*, for example, means "teacher." *Doctor*, derived from the Latin *doceo*, translates as "to lead and teach."

Maimonides' life and the prayer attributed to him emphasize the importance of ongoing learning by physicians and, by implication, recognize the significance of medical research in pushing the present boundaries of medical knowledge for the benefit of patients in the future: "Never allow the thought to arise in me that I have attained to sufficient knowledge, but vouchsafe to me the strength, the leisure and the ambition ever to extend my knowledge. For art is great, but the mind of man is ever expanding." Acting as a role model became equally important. From a Jewish perspective, these ideals are embraced by all physicians, particularly those engaged in academic medical settings, who pursue new discoveries and gain the wisdom that comes with experience to contextualize new knowledge for patient care through scholarly studies, research, and teaching.

The Ultimate Nature and Essential Concerns of Human Beings

Traditional Jews may ground their arguments in theology and reasoning differently from liberal Jews, who may focus more on universal existential concerns. Yet most Jews share a common set of values. The historian of religion Mircea Eliade observed that throughout human history, most cultures have identified a central core as the pinion for cultural life, order, and values. He terms this the *axis mundi*, the grounded center of existence. The Jewish axis mundi is the concept of Torah and the values that emanate from its long-held expression. Our journey in this chapter has helped us identify and reinforce the core elements that have shaped and manifested themselves in our professional practices. Eliade's observation is universal, suggesting that just as we have unearthed the origins, nature, and contexts of our core from a common source, every physician might benefit from such a personal journey that identifies, grounds, and propels the choice to become a doctor. Once so centered, the physician might find it easier to care for the well-being of others, to advocate for what is right and just, and to withstand the many demands, expectations, and challenges posed by the practice of medicine in the 21st century. Irrespective of differing cultural, religious, and faith traditions, we recommend our journey to others.

APPENDIX

The Prayer of Maimonides

Reproduced from Friedenwald 1917

> Almighty God, Thou hast created the human body with infinite wisdom. Ten thousand times ten thousand organs hast Thou combined in it that act unceasingly and harmoniously to preserve the whole in all its beauty—the body which is the envelope of the immortal soul. They are ever acting in perfect order, agreement and accord. Yet, when the frailty of matter or the unbridling of passions deranges this order or interrupts this accord, then the forces clash and the body crumbles

into the primal dust from which it came. Thou sendest to man diseases as beneficent messengers to foretell approaching danger and to urge him to avert it.

Thou hast blest Thine earth, Thy rivers and Thy mountains with healing substances; they enable Thy creatures to alleviate their sufferings and to heal their illnesses. Thou hast endowed man with the wisdom to relieve the suffering of his brother, to recognize his disorders, to extract the healing substances, to discover their powers and to prepare and to apply them to suit every ill. In Thine Eternal Providence Thou hast chosen me to watch over the life and health of Thy creatures. I am now about to apply myself to the duties of my profession. Support me, Almighty God, in these great labors that they may benefit mankind, for without Thy help not even the least thing will succeed.

Inspire me with love for my art and for Thy creatures. Do not allow thirst for profit, ambition for renown and admiration, to interfere with my profession, for these are the enemies of truth and of love for mankind and they can lead astray in the great task of attending to the welfare of Thy creatures. Preserve the strength of my body and of my soul that they ever be ready to cheerfully help and support rich and poor, good and bad, enemy as well as friend. In the sufferer let me see only the human being. Illumine my mind that it recognize what presents itself and that it may comprehend what is absent or hidden. Let it not fail to see what is visible, but do not permit it to arrogate to itself the power to see what cannot be seen, for delicate and indefinite are the bounds of the great art of caring for the lives and health of Thy creatures. Let me never be absent-minded. May no strange thoughts divert my attention at the bedside of the sick, or disturb my mind in its silent labors, for great and sacred are the thoughtful deliberations required to preserve the lives and health of Thy creatures.

Grant that my patients have confidence in me and my art and follow my directions and my counsel. Remove from their midst all charlatans and the whole host of officious relatives and know-all nurses, cruel people who arrogantly frustrate the wisest purposes of our art and often lead Thy creatures to their death.

Should those who are wiser than I wish to improve and instruct me, let my soul gratefully follow their guidance; for vast is the extent of our art. Should conceited fools, however, censure me, then let love for my profession steel me against them, so that I remain steadfast without regard for age, for reputation, or for honor, because surrender would bring to Thy creatures sickness and death.

Imbue my soul with gentleness and calmness when older colleagues, proud of their age, wish to displace me or to scorn me or disdainfully to teach me. May even this be of advantage to me, for they know many things of which I am ignorant, but let not their arrogance give me pain. For they are old and old age is not master of the passions. I also hope to attain old age on this earth, before Thee, Almighty God!

Let me be contented in everything except in the great science of my profession. Never allow the thought to arise in me that I have attained to sufficient knowledge, but vouchsafe to me the strength, the leisure and the ambition ever to extend my knowledge. For art is great, but the mind of man is ever expanding.

Almighty God! Thou hast chosen me in Thy mercy to watch over the life and death of Thy creatures. I now apply myself to my profession. Support me in this great task so that it may benefit mankind, for without Thy help not even the least thing will succeed.

REFERENCES

Eliade, M. 1959. *Cosmos and History: The Myth of the Eternal Return*. New York: Harper Torchbooks.

Friedenwald, H. 1917. Oath and prayer of Maimonides. *Bulletin of the Johns Hopkins Hospital* 28:260–61.

CHAPTER FOUR

Hinduism

Gowri Anandarajah, M.D.

Hinduism is as much a philosophy and a way of life as a religion. As such, it has a tremendous impact on the way millions of people worldwide view health, wellness, and science. It is the oldest living religion, dating back 10,000 years, according to astronomical verification of dates of events in scripture (Pandit 1993). There is no single founder of Hinduism; rather, it is inspired by divine revelation and is the product of the accumulated wisdom of the ancient sages and seers (*rishis*) of India, as well as that of the many saints who have come after them. The primary scriptures of Hinduism are the Vedas, which are said to have been revealed to the ancient rishis during deep meditation. These divine songs were transmitted orally for thousands of years and finally compiled into the four Vedas.

The real name for Hinduism is *Sanatana Dharma*, which roughly translated means "Eternal or Universal Righteousness." This name, plus its ancient origins, provides an important clue to the role this religion plays in the daily lives of Hindus. The significance of everyday events and action is interpreted within a framework that attempts to be universal in its scope and eternal in its time frame. Hinduism is a living, breathing religion that tries to make sense of apparent opposites and to provide guidance through the complexities of life. Thus, modern Hindus routinely try to bridge the distance between opposites: ancient versus modern, unity versus diversity, personal versus transpersonal, free will versus determinism. This becomes especially apparent when dealing with the issues surrounding suffering, illness, and death that we encounter daily in the practice of medicine.

As with any great world religion, whole textbooks are devoted to the subject of Hinduism. Also, as with other religions, numerous schools of thought, scriptures, and scholarly debates are to be found in the literature. It is beyond the scope of this chapter to do justice to the complexity that Hinduism encompasses. Rather, this chapter will outline some of the common concepts found in Hindu (Vedic) philosophy from the perspective of a Hindu physician with no formal training as a Vedic scholar but with strong academic interest in the subject of spirituality and medicine. I hope that this introduction provides a starting place from which physicians and other health care professionals can gain a better understanding of the role of Hinduism in the lives of patients and of professionals.

Basic Concepts of Hinduism

Aum, the Eternal Sound

> Aum. This eternal Word is all: what was, what is and what shall be, and what beyond is in eternity. All is Aum.
>
> MANDUKA UPANISHAD (MASCARO 1965, P. 83)

When people think of a Hindu, they often picture a thin, scantily dressed, cross-legged guru, sitting on the top of a mountain chanting "Aum." Although this stereotype is simplistic at best, many Hindus would argue that *Aum* (or Om) is the beginning, middle, and end of Hinduism. Thus, it is fitting to begin any discussion of Hinduism with an understanding of Aum. Aum is "God in sound," "the vibrational energy of the universe."

It is said that at the creation of the universe, the first creation was the sound (or word) "Aum." With this vibrational energy, the whole of creation came into being, and to this day Aum pervades every aspect of the universe. When we chant "Aum," we attune ourselves to the rest of the universe and to God. Because of this, Aum is the most powerful and most ancient mantra or prayer in Hinduism.

The Nature of God

Hindus believe in the existence of God. God is described as the "One Supreme Absolute" and beyond the comprehension of the human mind (which evolved for survival in the physical world). The name for this supreme reality is *Brahman*, whose chief attributes are *Sat* (infinite being), *Chit* (infinite awareness), and *Ananda* (infinite bliss). Other attributes include Pure Divine Love, Energy of the Universe, Absolute Truth, Absolute Peace, and so on. God is perceived as being everywhere and in all things. If the universe and all beings are like fish in water, then God is like the water, above, below, inside, and outside. God is also thought of as encompassing all apparent opposites—formless and in all forms, male and female, manifest and unmanifest.

Hinduism acknowledges that it is difficult for most people to relate to a formless God; it therefore accepts that humans may need to relate to God with form and attributes. Thus, it is fine to picture God in the form of a parent, loving friend, or beloved child if this brings one closer to God. The key is to remember that the form is only an access point to the formless and infinite. The following Vedic prayer, known to even the humblest village priest, encapsulates this concept:

> O Lord, forgive three sins that are due to my human limitations;
> Thou are everywhere, but I worship you here;
> Thou art without form, but I worship you in these forms;
> Thou needest no praise, yet I offer you these prayers and salutations;
> Lord, forgive three sins due to my human limitations.
>
> (SMITH 1991, P. 83)

Therefore, Hinduism states that in Brahman, there is Saguana Brahman, God with attributes (personal), and Nirguna Brahman, God without attributes (transpersonal). Both are correct. In simple terms, then, Hinduism can be described as "polymorphic monotheism" or "one God, many forms." The oldest of the Vedas, the Rig Veda, says, "Truth is one, the wise call it by various names" (Rig Veda I.164.46 [Pandit 1993, p. 10]).

The Nature of Human Beings

> Believe me, my son, an invisible and subtle essence is the Spirit of the whole universe. That is Reality. That is Atman. *Thou art that.*
>
> CHANDOGYA UPANISHAD (MASCARO 1965, P. 118)

Although there are differing schools of thought regarding the relationship between God and human beings (dualism, modified dualism, and nondualism), Advaita Vedanta is one of the most popular and is especially well accepted among scientific and intellectual communities. Advaita Vedanta maintains that everything is God (nondualism or monism). Because God pervades the whole universe, all of nature is divine, and therefore human beings are divine. The human spirit, or *Atma*, is a spark of the divine flame, a ray of the sun, a wave on the ocean.

The problem is that, although we human beings have the capacity to realize our inherent divinity, most of us do not recognize our true nature. We are caught in the illusion (*maya*) that the world as we see it with our five senses is all that there is. We fail to see that God, with infinite energy and love, is not only close to us at all times but also part of the fabric of our essential being. This illusion of separateness causes great suffering. The goal of human existence, according to Hindu belief, is to achieve closeness to God and ultimately union with God (going from duality to unity, from separateness to oneness). This takes a process of evolution. Just as the human body has undergone evolution to get to where it is, the human soul or consciousness (the inner part of which is the Atma) is going through a process of evolution.

Reincarnation

> Worn-out garments are shed by the body;
> Worn-out bodies are shed by the dweller.
>
> BHAGAVAD GITA 2.22 (SMITH 1991, P. 63)

Hinduism recognizes that the evolution of the human consciousness can take a long time. In keeping with its "eternal" view of cosmology, Hinduism maintains that for an individual soul (or *jiva*) to evolve, it has to pass through a sequence of bodies. This concept is called reincarnation, or transmigration of the soul.

With each life it lives, the jiva has a chance to grow in wisdom and love and to cast off the veil of illusion (maya) that prevents it from recognizing that its very being (Atma) is Being itself. According to Hindu thought, the evolution of consciousness that occurs with the evolution from subhuman to human bodies is automatic. However, once the soul enters a human body, the soul reaches self-consciousness, and with this comes freedom, responsibility, and effort. So, human beings have to choose to move forward the process of their own spiritual evolution. We will continue on this cycle of birth, death, and rebirth until we reach the level of spiritual development at which we see the whole world as a manifestation of the divine (duality) and ultimately realize our true identity with God (unity).

The Law of Karma: Cause and Effect

Hindus freely acknowledge that it is impossible for us to understand why God created the universe in which we live (see the Rig Veda creation poem in the appendix to this chapter). There are many theories and stories: creation is an expression of Love; a great experiment; God's play (*Leela*). We all have our favorite way of thinking of this. I like to think of God as Love: God, who is Love, creates the illusion of duality (i.e., creates "the other" from the One) in order for Love to be freely expressed. Hindus generally agree that God created a universe that functions under certain laws of cause and effect in order to continue. The physical laws of cause and effect, as seen in science, apply to the world. An understanding of these physical laws is, to a large degree, within our grasp as human beings. The karmic laws of cause and effect apply to the spirit, consciousness, and moral life. These are only partially within our ability to comprehend.

According to the law of karma, we live in a totally fair and moral universe. Karma literally means "action" or "work." This action can be in the form of thoughts, words, or deeds. Because everything in the universe is interconnected, every action has a consequence. Every action sends out a ripple in the fabric of the universe and eventually comes back to us. Our present condition is a direct result of past actions in this life or a past life. To complicate matters, karmic consequences can be linked to individual, family, or group actions. Because most of us have not reached a level of cosmic consciousness, we are not aware of everything that has happened in present and past lives and cannot figure out why exactly things happen the way they happen. Therefore, most Hindus will take the leap of faith and accept that there is meaning in what they encounter in daily life, even if they do not understand the reasons.

The law of karma accepts that our current situation is determined by the past (determinism). However, this law also maintains that we have the ability to influence our future by our present decisions, wants, and actions (free will). We are dealt a particular hand in a game of cards, but we are free to play the hand however we like. Therefore, because humans are self-conscious, by choosing what ripples we send out into the universe through our thoughts, words, and deeds, we actively participate in the creation of the future and in our own spiritual development. Mahatma Gandhi thought of it this way: "Although I believe in the inexorable law of karma, I am striving to do so many things; every moment of my life is a strenuous endeavor, which attempts to build up more karma, to undo the past and add to the present. It is therefore wrong to say that because my past is good, good is happening at present. The past would soon be exhausted, and I have to build up the future with prayer. I tell you karma alone is powerless" (Gandhi 2000, p. 38).

In summary, Hindus tend to accept that things happen for a reason. However, there is considerable individual variability in the degree to which people actively think about or worry about the concept of karma. In the medical setting, when patients are dealing with illness and death, the question of meaning can often arise. Because of the tremendous individual variability in outlook, it is generally best to ask open-ended questions to glean whether an individual's interpretation of karma is providing comfort or distress in these circumstances.

Dharma: Right Action

Hinduism provides guidelines regarding how people can generate positive, as opposed to negative, karma. These guidelines are encapsulated in the concept of dharma. Whole books are dedicated to the understanding of dharma; however, a brief introduction to the concept will be helpful to readers of this chapter. There is no direct English translation of the Sanskrit word *dharma*. However, approximations include "right action," "righteousness," "moral code," "doing the right thing," and "spiritual duty." We all have our spiritual duty (dharma), depending on our current circumstances, talents, and particular situation in life. It is our responsibility to figure out what our particular dharma is and then to act in accordance with it. We cannot judge or act on the dharma of others because only they are uniquely qualified to determine what is the "right" course of action for them. Although Hinduism gives guidelines regarding duties at various stages of life (student, householder, retiree, renunciant [one who renounces all worldly attachments]) and ethical principles (e.g., nonviolence, the ten major virtues, etc.), these guidelines do not take the place of individual responsibility for self-assessment and appropriate action. Underlying the concept of dharma is the principle of unity: we are all one, thus connected to and responsible for each other.

The Cause and Role of Suffering

In health care settings, we are confronted with suffering every day. This suffering takes physical, mental, and spiritual forms. As physicians, we are charged with the duty to alleviate this suffering to the best of our ability. Hinduism, like all other world religions, tries to provide a framework within which to view the meaning of suffering.

According to mainstream Hindu thought, physical suffering is a result of the physical and karmic laws of nature. Spiritual suffering, however, is due to identifying oneself as only the body and not drawing on the strength and comfort that come with identifying oneself with Spirit or God.

The reason that suffering exists is hard to fathom. Philosophers, poets, and religious scholars from all over the world have struggled with this question for thousands of years. If God is all-knowing, all-powerful, and all-loving, why would God allow suffering to exist? In Hinduism there are many perspectives on this question.

One perspective from Hindu thought that might shed light on this question stems from the idea that human spiritual development occurs by overcoming suffering and the limitations of the physical body and mind. By overcoming suffering, one is able to see what lies beyond what is immediately apparent and start a process of spiritual transformation. Because the world will always have pleasure and pain, the goal is to put these in perspective and be unaffected by or detached from either (equanimity). This does not mean that one cannot fully participate in life; it just means that events are viewed in a broader context. As we become less attached to the world of pleasure and pain, we have the opportunity to become more attached to the Transcendent, to God.

Hindus believe that God has the power to suspend the laws of nature to intervene in human events (and sometimes may do this, through Grace). However, if God did this routinely, the universe (which functions according to the laws of cause and effect) would come to a grinding halt. Evolution and human spiritual development would also stop. God's role is similar to that of the parent in the following analogy: A parent, watching a child learn how to walk, is moved by compassion and provides pillows to soften the child's falls. The parent resists the temptation to carry the child around all the time, because he or she knows that unless the child is allowed to try and fall, the child will never learn to walk. Similarly, God will be moved by compassion to lighten the burden and soften the falls whenever possible, but will allow human spiritual development to continue. This idea is expressed in a line from a devotional song: "Let the pain I have to bear be light." God also relieves suffering through the actions of mankind. This idea is encapsulated by Mahatma Gandhi: "God does not come down in person to relieve suffering. He works through human agency. Therefore, prayer to God, to enable one to relieve the suffering of others, must mean a longing and readiness on one's part to labor for it" (Gandhi 2000, p. 35).

What Do You Want?

> Even as the unwise work selfishly in the bondage of selfish works, let the wise man work unselfishly for the good of all the world.
>
> BHAGAVAD GITA 3:25 (MASCARO 1962, P. 58)

Hinduism accepts that people are different. We are different in our personality types, abilities, and affinities; we are different in our backgrounds and place of origin; and we are different in our starting point on the spiritual path. To understand why people are at different starting points on the spiritual path, Hinduism provides a framework within which to understand people's motivations and degree of active interest in spirituality. Because once the soul (or jiva) enters the human body, further spiritual evolution requires self-effort, the answer to the question "What do you want?" helps determine the degree and type of spiritual growth that will occur during that lifetime.

Hinduism asserts that people basically want four things. They start by wanting pleasure. This is natural, and as long as one observes the basic rules of morality, Hinduism accepts that this is a legitimate goal of life for many people. People can happily spend a large portion of their life or multiple lifetimes pursuing pleasure. However, Hinduism also asserts that eventually people grow tired of momentary pleasures, and their focus will then shift to the second major goal of life, which is worldly success (wealth, fame, and power).

Worldly success is also a reasonable goal of life. It requires putting off some immediate pleasure for longer-term satisfaction. Although a certain degree of worldly success is necessary for supporting a household and discharging civic duties, Hinduism states that eventually this too can lose its appeal. This is because the desire for individual success can never be fully satisfied. With success, one can always envision ways to become more famous, wealthy, and powerful. Individual success also often involves competing with others, which can lead to fear that one is on precarious ground, never sure of when wealth, fame, or power will be lost. Eventually, the desire for worldly success loses its appeal, and people start looking around for something more. Hinduism, with its long-term perspective, accepts that it may take the soul (jiva) several lifetimes to get to the point at which it starts searching for more.

Once a person realizes that he or she is on an endless treadmill chasing after desires that will never be satisfied, the person starts looking around for meaning beyond individual pleasure and success. At this point, the person turns toward the third major goal in life, service to community. The focus is shifted from one's own individual needs to the needs of the greater community.

Hinduism outlines many ways in which one can perform one's duties to society suitable to age, temperament, and social status. This search for meaning and value beyond the individual self is the first step in leading a spiritual, or dharmic, life. However, Hinduism states that even this stage, with its focus on the well-being of the community, eventually loses its driving appeal because it is limited to the physical world, to history, and to time.

Eventually, people start wondering if there is more to life than pleasure, success, and service to society. This can be triggered by certain powerful experiences, including suffering, or may flow as a natural consequence of several lifetimes spent in the pursuit of the first three goals of life. Once an individual begins an active line of questioning involving life, death, meaning, and purpose, Hinduism asserts that the part of human beings that is infinite (the Atma) drives us to yearn for a goal in life that is beyond the scope of the world as we see it. The thing that Hinduism states people want more than anything else is God, union with the Infinite and liberation from the endless cycle of birth and death (*moksha*). When people start to realize that this is what they really want, they start serious exploration of the various paths to God.

Pathways for Spiritual Development: The Four Yogas

In keeping with its assertion that people are different, Hinduism accepts that there are many possible paths in our journeys to God. Depending on their personality type, abilities, and life situation, people are often better suited to certain paths than to others. A frequently cited analogy is that of climbing a mountain. The goal is to reach the top of the mountain (i.e., God). There are many possible paths up the mountain, some challenging, steep but direct, some less challenging but longer. However, the goal for all paths is the same. At the base of the mountain, the paths look different. However, near the top of the mountain, the paths begin to converge.

Because of this view of diverse spiritual paths, mainstream Hinduism is accepting of different approaches to spiritual growth. Modern Hindus will generally agree that all the major world religions teach valid paths toward God. There is no need to convert from one religion to another. What is necessary is to dig deep in the spiritual tradition for which you have the greatest affinity. The first step on all meaningful paths is the cultivation of basic human values such as truth, right conduct, peace, love, and nonviolence.

Hinduism describes four basic types of pathways for spiritual growth—the four Yogas. The meaning of the word *yoga* is not limited to the common Western understanding of yoga, which are the exercises seen in Hatha Yoga. A yoga is a method of training that leads to the union of the human spirit to God. The four Yogas are Jnana Yoga (the Path of Knowledge), Bhakthi Yoga (the Path of Love), Karma Yoga (the Path of Work), and Raj Yoga (the Royal Path). People may use one path predominantly or a combination of paths in their spiritual journey.

The Path of Knowledge (Jnana Yoga)

Jnana Yoga is best suited for those people who possess strong intellectual and reflective ability and combine this with a deep longing for God. The knowledge that this path requires is not just book knowledge but wisdom and intuitive discernment—the ability to distinguish illusion from truth. It is the shortest but steepest path because it requires this rare combination of rationality and spirituality.

There are generally three stages in this path. The first is listening to the scriptures, sages, prophets, and gurus. This introduces the seeker to the idea that his or her essential being is Being itself. Second comes thinking. Through a process of intense contemplation and reflection on the concept of unity between the Atma and God, the Atma (God within) changes from concept to realization. Several exercises are used to achieve this shift, similar to the koans seen in Zen Buddhism. One example is reflection on the word *my* ("my book," "my body," "my mind"). Who is the "I" who possesses the body and the mind? It is the witness, the unchanging Atma. The third stage consists of shifting self-identification from the limited, mortal body/mind/ego to the unlimited, expansive Atma/God. This final step is extremely challenging but will ultimately lead to self-realization. In this state of cosmic consciousness, the jnana yogi can still function "in the world" but is not "of the world" and may act as a guide for other seekers.

The Path of Love (Bhakti Yoga)

> He who in this oneness of love, loves Me in whatever he sees, wherever this man may live, in truth this man lives in Me.
>
> BHAGAVAD GITA 6:31 (MASCARO 1962, P. 71)

The Path of Love is the most popular of the four yogas because emotion and love are something most people can relate to. This is a well-worn, wide path with a gradual ascent up the mountain. To the bhakti yogi, feelings are more real than thought. The yogi sees God as personal rather than transpersonal. The goal is not to be God but rather to love God with every element of one's being—maintaining some degree of duality. "I want to taste the sugar; I don't want to be the sugar" (Smith, 1991). The love the bhakti yogi feels is love for love's sake with no ulterior motives. As affection for God increases, the world's grip on us decreases. Saints do love the world, but in a different way from others. They see it as a reflection of God's glory. Modern Hindus would view Christianity as an example of an important bhakti highway to God.

Because of the bhakti yogi's need for a personal connection with God, and the tremendous variability between individual human beings, Hinduism embraces the idea that God, who is formless and in all forms, can be visualized in many different forms. The idea is that God can become available to the seeker in whatever form helps the seeker relate to God. This enhances one's ability to love God more deeply.

This concept of God as accessible through form is where Hinduism's numerous images of gods and goddesses enter the picture. Each god or goddess represents an aspect of the One Supreme Absolute, and each has attributes that can help seekers along their spiritual path. Hinduism has a rich mythology that brings to life these gods and goddesses and provides stories that illustrate the ways in which one can live a good life. This is a living mythology that is very much a part of the modern-day Hindu's psyche. In India, images of God can be seen everywhere. Artistic renditions of the gods and goddesses of Hindu mythology are found not only in temples but also in statues and artwork in buildings and parks and in pictures on simple altars in corners of stores and in taxicabs. Most Hindus, even those living in Western countries, have altars in their homes and at work. Hindus on the bhakti path usually choose a particular form of God as a focus for worship. This chosen form is their entry point to the formless, and it is clearly understood that one must worship the image as if it were God, not God as if it were the image.

Many different methods are used for devotion or worship on the bhakti path. *Japam* is the repeating of God's name—"keep the name of the Lord spinning in the midst of all your daily activities" (Smith 1991, p. 35). *Bhajans*, or devotional songs, are used for individual and group devotion. Mantras are prescribed words, phrases, or verses from scripture that when recited enhance the ability of the mind to contemplate the divine. Rituals are frequently performed in the temple and at home. Many use individual prayer and meditation on a daily basis. Pilgrimages to holy places—"where so many have worshiped with Love, God is truly present" (unknown author)—and seeking the *darshan* (blessing) of holy people (saints), who embody God's energy more strongly than others, are other methods of devotion. Famous bhakti yogis from different world religions include Sri Ramakrishnan, Meerabai, Rumi, and St. John of the Cross.

In the hospital setting, it is often difficult for patients to access the methods of worship that usually bring them a sense of inner peace and connection with God. Through simple open-ended inquiry, health care professionals can help patients and families access their own personal spiritual resources, such as bringing in God pictures for the bedside table or tapes of devotional songs to which they can listen when alone.

The Path of Work (Karma Yoga)

> This man of harmony surrenders the reward of his work and thus attains final peace: the man of disharmony, urged by desires, is attached to his reward and remains in bondage. BHAGAVAD GITA 5:12 (MASCARO 1962, P. 67)

Karma Yoga (or selfless service) is the path that is the most suited to people who are active. For most people, work or action is a necessary part of life.

The Path of Work maintains that one can grow spiritually in the world of everyday activities, without the need to withdraw from society to be with God. The method of doing this yoga depends on the worker's primary nature: affective or reflective. For those who have a primarily affective nature, karma yoga is performed in the bhakti (devotion) mode. Those who have a more reflective nature can perform karma yoga in the jnana (knowledge) mode.

For Karma Yoga in the bhakti mode, the yogi sees God in everyone and everything. Therefore, service to others is service to God. Action is performed out of love alone, without attachment to the results. The motivation behind the action is important: it must be selfless, with no trace of selfishness. The true yogi has no desire for personal rewards such as recognition, thanks, fame, or fortune and considers it to be God's energy that is working through him or her to produce good work: "Thou art the doer, I am the instrument" (Smith 1991). When the yogi does work with this attitude, each act in life becomes an act of service and a form of worship. When a person surrenders the fruits of all action to God, the world begins to loose its grip on the individual and the yogi grows in spiritual love for both the world and God. Gradually the yogi pays off his or her accumulated karmic debt without adding new negative deeds to his or her karmic burden, and eventually reaches self-realization. Hindus would consider Mother Theresa and St. Francis of Assisi to be excellent examples of karma yogis in bhakti mode.

The jnana approach to karma yoga is based on the idea that work is performed in detachment from the empirical self and in identity with the eternal. The yogi sees the whole world as being interconnected and "One." Because of this point of view, it makes sense that work should be done keeping in mind what is best for the whole. Work is done as part of one's dharmic responsibility, because it is the "right thing to do." As with the bhakti mode, the yogi remains indifferent to the personal consequences of the actions. This leads to decreased ego and decreased selfishness. Mahatma Gandhi is an example of someone who often functioned in this mode.

According to Hindu philosophy, it is also possible for someone to be a karma yogi without believing in any particular religion or religious doctrine. Selfless service performed for the right reasons (e.g., out of compassion or because it is the "right thing to do") with no thought of personal reward will automatically generate positive karma, reduce karmic debt, and eventually lead to salvation.

The Path of Psychophysical Exercises (Raj Yoga)

> Day after day, let the yogi practice the harmony of the soul: in a secret place, in deep solitude, master of his mind, hoping for nothing, desiring nothing.
>
> BHAGAVAD GITA 6:10 (MASCARO 1962, P. 70)

Raj Yoga leads to union with God through the expansion of human consciousness using a systematic process involving psychophysical exercises. This is a rigorous path that is best suited for people who have an affinity for scientific methodology and self-discipline. The various exercises in this path were developed by the ancient rishis of India over thousands of years. They performed experiments in consciousness expansion on themselves, carefully recorded results, and passed on their findings to their disciples, who further developed the techniques. By this process, the rishis systematically charted a course through human consciousness that can be replicated under the personal guidance of a high-quality teacher (or guru). Because advanced techniques can be treacherous unless learned under proper guidance, it is essential that one choose one's guru wisely. One would not want to climb Mount Everest without the help of an experienced guide who knows the best paths that avoid the dangerous chasms. The same caution should apply to climbing through the levels of human consciousness.

The practice of Raj Yoga prepares the body and mind for perfect concentration. Perfect concentration leads to perfect meditation, which ultimately leads to the superconscious state (*samadhi*) in which one is united with the ultimate reality. There are eight steps in this yogic discipline: Yama (moral and ethical discipline), Niyama (spiritual observances), Asana (body posture), Pranayama (breath control), Pratyahara (withdrawing the mind from sense perception), Dharna (concentration), Dhyana (meditation), and Samadhi (union with God).

It is beyond the scope of this chapter to review each of these steps in detail. However, it is important to note that true meditation (dhyana) is not a particular action that one performs. Rather, it is a spontaneous phenomenon that occurs when the mind is in a thoughtless state of nondoing.

In this state, one has access to the vast untapped wisdom that is present in oneself (the Atma). Samadhi occurs spontaneously when the yogi is in a state of deep meditation and has several levels. These levels range from conscious samadhi, to superconscious samadhi (communion with God) with body attachment, to superconscious samadhi without body attachment (i.e., oneness with God).

Many techniques can be used to develop perfect concentration that allows meditation to occur spontaneously. Among these are such things as focusing on a mantra (word or phrase), on an image of God, on one's own breath, or on a part of the body.

Hatha Yoga is a branch of Raj Yoga that is popular throughout the world as a way to maintain the health and vitality of the body and mind. The yogis of India learned early on that certain body postures and regulated breathing helped prepare the mind for focusing inward. Thus, the simple practice of the postures in Hatha Yoga (such as the sun salutation) can at least improve physical and mental health and at best prepare one for spiritual growth through meditation.

Laya Yoga and Tantric Yoga are variations of Raj Yoga which are generally followed by those who have an understanding of the energy centers of the body (the seven chakras) and the ways energy flows through the body from kundalini energy stored at the base of the spine to the higher energy centers in the body. In these yogic practices, the yogi gradually causes the latent kundalini energy to rise up the energy channels located in the spinal canal, progressively activating each of the chakras. When kundalini energy finally reaches the last chakra at the top of the head, the yogi enters the superconscious state of samadhi and union with God.

The above discussion is a brief overview of the various approaches Hindus might use in their quest for the divine. Due to the huge variations in human nature and degree of active interest in spirituality, it is important for clinicians to approach their patients as individuals. Yoga philosophy is a useful framework through which clinicians can begin to better understand a particular patient's spiritual needs.

A Note on Ayurvedic Medicine

Although this chapter is focused on Hindu beliefs and values that may inform the care of Hindu patients in the context of the practice of Western medicine, this chapter would be incomplete without at least a brief mention of Ayurvedic medicine. Ayurvedic medicine is a complete system of medicine that is based on the Vedic literature. This ancient system of medicine (developed in 1000–500 BCE) is still practiced in many countries worldwide and employs multiple treatment approaches, including herbal medications, surgical interventions, massage therapy, breath control, yoga postures, and meditation. Diagnosis and treatment approaches are based on a holistic view of the human being as being composed of five "sheaths" and three "bodies." The physical body includes the gross body sheath (e.g., anatomy, physiology, biochemistry) and the energy body sheath (prana energy, chakras, kundalini). The subtle body includes the lower mind sheath (thoughts and emotion) and the higher mind sheath (intellect and wisdom). The causal body comprises the bliss sheath, which includes the Atma (spirit).

Ayurvedic treatment focuses on bringing into balance the three body types, or *doshas*, inherent in every person—Vata, Pitta, and Kapha. Hindus as well as other patients from around the world may use Ayurvedic medicine in addition to allopathic medicine, so it is reasonable to inquire about this during the course of medical care.

Hinduism and Science

In Vedanta philosophy, the universe is seen as being infused with God, and human beings are expected to seek knowledge and understanding. Because of this, the exploration of the universe through scientific methods is seen as a valid way to learn more about ourselves, the world around us, and ultimately God. Because science deals with the outer world—the world that can be perceived and measured using the five senses—it provides important but limited information about the universe. Therefore, Hinduism asserts that a complete understanding of reality requires a combination of both scientific and spiritual inquiry. This comfort with science has permitted devout Hindus throughout the world to pursue careers in every major scientific field and in general allows Hindu patients to be comfortable with scientific approaches to medical care.

The Medical Care of the Hindu Patient

This chapter presented some basic concepts in Hinduism that may be helpful in the medical care of Hindu patients. The following is a summary and a few simple guidelines for patient care.

1. Hindus vary tremendously in their approach to spirituality and to life, so approach people as individuals and use the information in this chapter as a framework within which to understand a particular patient. It is also important to be aware of potential differences in

the degrees to which Hindus have been immersed in the culture and philosophy of Hinduism, depending on whether they were raised in India or a Western country.

2. In general, Hindus believe in God. However, they visualize God in many different ways and vary in the degrees in which God is a part of their daily lives. If a patient visualizes God as a personal God (friend, mother, father, etc.), illness and suffering can trigger strong emotions directed at God, ranging from anger and fear to an intense yearning for love. Identifying when this is happening and providing understanding and resources to help can assist in the healing process.
3. A patient may use a variety of spiritual resources to help during difficult times. Use open-ended questions to find out what is most important to the patient personally. Because many people use the bhakti path, it may help to inquire specifically about rituals, methods of worship (e.g., prayer, bhajan, meditation), or practices (e.g., a vegetarian diet) that may be important to each person.
4. In general, Hindus believe in an afterlife. The concept of karma and rebirth may influence the way they approach treatment decisions, including end-of-life decisions. An individual's interpretation of karmic consequences could result in spiritual distress for some and spiritual peace for others. If it appears that a patient is distressed over questions regarding meaning, it is important to explore further.
5. For many Hindus, religious factors and cultural factors overlap tremendously. In caring for Hindu patients, one must keep in mind the importance of family and family elders in critical medical decision making. It is possible that a patient may want to defer to the wisdom of a family elder regarding the dharmic ("right") course of action.

Personal Reflections

Hindu philosophy helps ground me in many ways. As a Hindu growing up in Western countries, I vividly remember a time in elementary school (a British, Christian school) when the concept that there was one God, accessible through many paths, opened up the whole world to me. I could fully participate in all school religious activities and could freely learn about all the world's religions, including my own. Hinduism's acceptance of science supported my curiosity regarding seeking truth through scientific exploration.

I wish I could say that I am spiritually enlightened enough to have chosen a career in medicine as a conscious step along my spiritual path. I am not! However, given that I stumbled into academic family medicine as much out of luck (perhaps karma?) as by anything else, it has been a great path for me. The practice of medicine puts us on the front lines of human experience. We get to be witnesses to it all—the joys of birth and the intense sorrow of untimely death. We hear the first-hand stories of people from all walks of life—their struggles, their resources, their hopes, and their fears. I have been humbled by the incredible resilience of some of my patients who have overcome intensely difficult life situations, and I have been inspired by the peace and courage with which some of my patients have approached death. In medicine we are given the daily opportunity to engage in the drama of life. Vedanta philosophy compels me to value my patients' various perspectives. While this helps me find the best ways to help them clinically, it also gives me the opportunity to let my patients be my teachers.

Hinduism also requires a certain degree of self-reflection, which keeps me from going too far off course. As an "action" person with a devotional bent, I am best suited to the karma yoga path in the bhakti mode. I have found that patient care and teaching are my best spiritual disciplines, as long as I remember that I am aspiring to perform selfless service and to see the good in even the most challenging person. I ask God almost every day for help with this! The question "What do you want?" reminds me to catch myself when I get too caught up in the hamster wheel (easy to do in academic medicine). I try to ask myself why I am choosing to do what I do: is it for my own desire for individual success, or is it out of a genuine sense of selfless service?

I have a long way to go along the spiritual path toward liberation, with many more lives left to go. However, I am grateful for this life—for my family and friends, my teachers, my students, my patients, my colleagues, and for the many opportunities God has given me to serve and to grow. Whenever I get discouraged, I remember the following quotation from my favorite modern-day spiritual teacher: "When the sun rises and shines, not all the lotus buds in the lakes and ponds bloom; only those that are ready, do. The rest have to bide their time. But all are destined to bloom; all have to fulfill that destiny. There is no need to despair" (Sri Sathya Sai Baba, quotation 26 in Baba 1985).

We'll all get there eventually. We just need faith, love, hope, and perseverance.

APPENDIX

The Creation Hymn of the Rig Veda

Translation from Panikkar 1977

At first was neither Being nor Nonbeing.
There was not air nor yet sky beyond.
What was wrapping? Where? In whose protection?
Was Water there, unfathomable deep?

There was no death then, nor yet deathlessness;
of night or day there was not any sign.
The One breathed without breath by its own impulse.
Other than that was nothing at all.

Darkness was there, all wrapped around by darkness,
and all was Water indiscriminate, Then
that which was hidden by Void, that One, emerging,
stirring, through power of Ardor, came to be.

In the beginning Love arose,
which was primal germ cell of mind.
The Seers, searching in their hearts with wisdom,
discovered the connection of Being in Nonbeing.

A crosswise line cut Being from Nonbeing.
What was described above it, what below?
Bearers of seed there were and mighty forces,
thrust from below and forward move above.

Who really knows? Who can presume to tell it?
Whence was it born? Whence issued this creation?
Even the gods came after its emergence.
Then who can tell from whence it came to be?

That, out of which creation has arisen,
whether it held it firm or it did not,
He who surveys it in the highest heaven,
He surely knows—or maybe He does not!

REFERENCES

Arya, P. P. 1999. *Sai Baba and Moksha*. Delhi: Professional Media House.
Baba, S. S. 1985. *One Single Stream of Love*. Puttaparthi, India: Sri Sathya Sai Books.
Crossman, K. 2002. *Selections from the Gospel of Sri Ramakrishna; Annotated and Explained.* Woodstock, VT: Skylights Path Publishing.

Desai, P. N. 1989. *Health and Medicine in the Hindu Tradition*. New York: Crossroad.
Doniger, W., trans. 1981. *The Rig Veda*. London: Penguin.
Gandhi, M. K. 2000. *Prayer.* Ed. John Strohmeier. Berkeley: Berkeley Hills Books.
Harvey, A. 1996. *The Essential Mystics*. New York: Harper San Francisco.
Lad, V. 2002. *Textbook of Ayurveda*, vol. 1: *Fundamental Principles*. Albuquerque, NM: Ayurvedic Press.
Mascaro, J., trans. 1962. *The Bhagavad Gita*. London: Penguin.
———, trans. 1965. *The Upanishads*. London: Penguin.
Pandit, B. 1993. *The Hindu Mind: Fundamentals of Hindu Religion and Philosophy for All Ages*. Illinois: B & V Enterprises.
Panikkar, R. 1977. *The Vedic Experience—Mantra-manjari: An Anthology of the Vedas for Modern Man and Contemporary Celebration*. Delhi, India: Motilal Banarasidas. Mountain Man's Global News Archive, 1997. www.mountainman.com.au/news97_8.html. Accessed 25 Aug. 2009.
Smith, H. 1991. *The World's Religions: Our Great Wisdom Traditions*. New York: HarperCollins.

CHAPTER FIVE

Islam

Areej El-Jawahri, M.D.

Islam is a monotheistic religion that was established in 610 CE by the Prophet Muhammad. Currently, more than 1.2 billion people identify as Muslims. Forty percent of Muslims are Asians originating from India, Pakistan, Afghanistan, Indonesia, Malaysia, China, and the Philippines; 20 percent are from the Middle East (including non-Arab countries Iran and Turkey); 30 percent are from sub-Saharan Africa; 3 percent are native to Europe; and 1 percent are native to the Americas. Islam is the fastest-growing religion in North America; there are more than 3 million Muslims in the United States.

The Ultimate Nature and Essential Concerns of Human Beings

The word *Islam* in Arabic translates to "submission to the will of God" (Allah). The root of the word *Islam* stems from the Arabic word *salam*, which means "peace," signifying the importance of peace in Islam. For an individual Muslim, Islam becomes the path to allow a person to reach inner peace with him- or herself, with the Creator (Allah), and with creation. This can be accomplished only by complete and utter surrender to the will of God. Islam acknowledges many prophets as the messengers of God who were sent to guide humankind. These prophets include figures such as Adam, David, Solomon, Noah, Abraham, Moses, and Jesus. Muslims believe in angels, heaven and hell, and the Day of Judgment. They believe that Jesus will return to Jerusalem before the Day of Judgment. They believe that Mary (who is mentioned more times in the Quran than in the New Testament) had a virgin conception—that her pregnancy was a miracle—but not that Jesus was the son of God. They believe in large passages of the Torah (Jewish scripture) and the Old Testament. The holy book for Muslims, the Quran, was revealed to the last prophet and messenger of God, Muhammad.

God upholds the integrity of every existing being. God alone is an infinite and original being. God created nature for humans to exploit and use for good purposes. Numerous verses in the Quran proclaim that God has "made subservient the heaven and the earth and whatever is in them to humankind." According to the Quran, the fundamental weaknesses of humans are pettiness, narrow-mindedness, and selfishness. People should transcend these weaknesses by self-giving to others. Faith bestows safety and peace, and by accepting and surrendering to the law of God, which is the ultimate protection against perils, one avoids disintegration. Thus, Islam states that people should avoid moral and physical peril, conform to the law of God, and thus save themselves individually and collectively from perdition. In so doing, they develop their vast potential by obeying God's moral law.

For many, Islam is not just a religion but a way of life. There is a strong emphasis on families in Muslim societies. This includes not only includes immediate family members but also all blood relatives and the Islamic community, where a sense of brotherhood and sisterhood is an integral aspect of Muslim faith.

In the Muslim worldview, God gives rights that cannot be separated from duties toward the Creator and fellow human beings. For example, while all healing ultimately comes from God, Muslims have a duty to seek out medical attention when ill and a right to receive appropriate medical care. Physicians have a clear obligation to provide medical care. The reciprocity of rights and duties differs from the Western conception of inherent and inalienable rights.

Islam does not distinguish between religion and spirituality. There is no spirituality without religious thoughts, practice, and experience. Religion provides the spiritual path for salvation and a way of life. Muslims accept the Divine and seek meaning, purpose, and happiness in a worldly life and the hereafter. At the core of the Islamic system lies the practice of spiritual discipline, which educates and trains the inner person. It frees a person from the slavery of him- or herself, purges the soul from the lust of materialistic life, and instills in humans a tremendous love for God. Through patience, perseverance, and gratitude, one can open the door for spiritual and physical well-being. No matter how high a person's moral and spiritual station, he or she cannot take it for granted and feel immune; a person has always to try not to fall but to climb up.

For Muslims, earth is a resting place for the purpose of worshipping God and doing good deeds and for following one's duties toward the Creator, toward each other, and toward the surrounding environment. When asked what actions are most excellent, the Prophet Muhammad responded: "To gladden the hearts of human beings, to feed the hungry, to help the afflicted, to lighten the sorrow of the sorrowful, and to remove the suffering of the injured" (Sahih Bukhari, book 6; also in Ali 1983, p. 22). Muslims are also taught to accept death as a part of a journey, an end to a worldly life followed by a spiritual journey of a greater importance. "Wherever you are, death will find you out, even if you are in towers built up strong and high!" (Quran 4:78).

Insights about Life and Healing

> Seek treatment, because Allah did not send down a sickness but has sent down a medication for it—known to those who know it and not known to others except for death.
>
> THE PROPHET MUHAMMAD (SUNAN ABUDAWUD, BOOK 28, HADITH 3846)

> And when I am sick, then God restores me to health; and He it is who will cause me to die, then give me a life [in purgatory and again on the day of Judgment].
>
> QURAN 26:80–81

Central to Islamic teachings are the connections among knowledge, health, holism, the environment, and the oneness of God (i.e., the unity of God in all spheres of life, death, and the hereafter). Islamic teachings and practice provide a holistic framework for meeting the physical, spiritual, psychosocial, and environmental needs of individual and communities. Health and illness, life and death, are active realities in Islam. However, this does not negate the importance of seeking medical attention, practicing good health habits, and performing one's duty toward protecting the body. Human beings should be responsible stewards of their bodies, which are gifts from God. They have an obligation to protect the body and attend to its needs.

Pleasure and suffering in Islam are thought to be in God's hands, brought to humankind by the will of God. However, the meaning of suffering can be perceived differently by Muslims depending on their cultural background, family values, and level of education. Some Muslims perceive suffering as a way of atoning for sins. Others perceive illness as a natural occurrence and accept it as the will of God. The prophet stated, "No fatigue, nor disease, nor sorrow, nor sadness, nor hurt, nor distress befalls a Muslim, even if it were the prick he received from a thorn, but Allah expiates some of his sins for that" (Sahih Bukhari, book 70, Hadith 545). Still other Muslims perceive suffering as a test from God, but one that carries with it tidings of forgiveness and mercy: "Be sure we shall test you with something of fear, hunger, some loss in wealth, lives or the produce [of your soil], but give glad tidings to those who patiently persevere" (Quran 2:155).

Muslims are expected to receive illness with patience, meditation, and prayers—not necessarily as an enemy, but rather as an event, a mechanism of the body, that is serving to cleanse, purify, and balance the self on physical, emotional, mental, and spiritual planes: "Every human being is bound to taste Death, and we test you [all] through the bad and the good [things in life] by way of trial; and unto Us you all must return" (Quran 21:35).

Health and illness become part of the continuum of being, and prayer remains the salvation in both health and in sickness. The Prophet wrote, "The prayer of the sick person will never be rejected, until he recovers" (Rassool 2000, p. 1480).

The sayings and actions of the Prophet Mohammed, which are called Sunnah, fall into two categories with regard to medicine. Some encourage medical treatment in case of sickness and offer broad principles that promote health, while others are putative statements of the Prophet on particular diseases and health problems (including measures to treat them medically or spiritually). With respect to the first category, the Prophet focused on general principles, mostly preventive, that prohibit lifestyle and other behaviors that are hazardous to health, and prescribed behaviors that promote health: moderate eating; abstinence from alcohol, tobacco, and other substances; regular exercise; prayer; fasting; ablution and bathing; and breast feeding. The Quranic verse "Eat, drink, but do not commit excesses" (7:31), quoted by almost all writers, is regarded in Islam as the ultimate means for preventing sickness.

Islam also addresses psychosomatic illness. The Prophet Muhammad once stated, "Excessive worry makes for physical illness in a person," indicating his emphasis on attending to both psychological and spiritual health.

Islamic teachings encourage those in Muslim communities to visit the sick and provide support and comfort in difficult times. Numerous sayings of the Prophet exhort the faithful to visit the sick and give them hope and comfort: "Visit the sick and free captives" (Prophet Muhammad, Sahih Bukhan, book 52, Hadith 282). Abu Huraira, a favorite companion of the Prophet, reported him as saying, "God shall say on the Day of Judgment, 'O son of Adam! I was sick but you did not visit me.'" Man will reply, "My Lord! How could I visit you when you are the Lord of the whole world." God will then say, "Did you not know that so and so from among my servants [that is, human beings] was sick but you never visited him or her? Did you not know that if you had visited, you would have found me there?" (Rahman 1987, p. 59).

The mental, moral, and spiritual aspect of a physician's work is highly valued in Islam. After faith, the art and practice of medicine is the most meritorious service in God's sight, according to the Prophet Muhammad. The early-15th-century medical writer Al-Azraq writes in the introduction to *Medical Benefits Made Accessible*, "Medicine is a science whose benefits are great and whose nobility, prestige, and fame are recognized and whose roots are established in the Book [the Quran], and the Example [Sunna]."

It is the physician's duty to interrelate the spiritual and bodily health of the patient. Physicians should be cultured, should gain the trust of the patient, and should cultivate professional confidence. Physicians must be self-reliant and should never lose patience with their patients. Time should be given generously to the patient, and physicians should do more listening and less talking in the medical encounter. The Prophet states, "A physician should be of kindly disposition, characterized by rational thought and possessed of excellent intuitive power" (Rahman 1987, p. 38). Physicians are expected to provide care to the patient and the entire family. They are also expected to address existential issues pertaining to death and dying, deal with spiritual concerns, and alleviate psychological suffering.

Relationship to Contemporary Medical Practice

When discussing ethical dilemmas faced by Muslim patients in hospitals throughout the world, one must first consider Islamic law, with a particular focus on Islamic medical ethics. Islamic law or Islamic doctrine (Sharia), which provides guidance for all Muslims on how to behave on earth, stems from three main sources: the Quran, the saying and actions of the Prophet Mohammed (Sunnah), and the process of Ijtihad (the law of deductive logic), which charges Muslim jurists with interpreting and contextualizing religious teachings for the wider Muslim community (following principles such as law by analogy, law by consensus, etc.). Distinct schools of Islam have followers in different Muslim sects. When there is a disagreement among Muslim jurists with regard to a given legal question, Muslims are permitted to follow any of the scholars' views and not necessarily the view of their sect. However, generally speaking, Muslims feel strongly about following a particular school of Islamic thought.

Islamic medical ethics consist of four general principles. These are, in order of importance, nonmaleficence ("Do no harm"), justice, respect for patient autonomy, and beneficence. While these are similar to Western principles, Islamic ethics also place a primary focus on the preservation of one's faith through the illness, the sanctity of life, alleviation of suffering, enjoying what is good and permitted, and forbidding what is wrong and prohibited. The following pages summarize the Islamic perspective on some common dilemmas.

Modesty and Social Interactions

Modesty is a frequent point of tension for Muslim patients in Western society. Muslim male patients often prefer to be examined by male doctors, while Muslim women prefer to be examined by female doctors. Some Muslims take this to an extreme and consider it prohibited for one to be examined by a physician of the opposite gender. The Islamic religious stance on this is clear and agreed on by Muslim jurists. Islam allows opposite-gender health care providers to examine patients in private, primarily to show the utmost respect to the sacred physician-patient relationships that should transcend human desires and instincts. However, many Muslims in the general population are not aware of this stance. As discussed previously, culture, upbringing, and level of education play an important role in Muslims' overall understanding of their religion and application of their "religious" principles in daily life. Hence, this will continue to be an issue in taking care of Muslim patients.

Psychiatric Illness

Although classic Islamic teachings have promoted psychiatric health and psychological well-being, psychiatric illness continues to carry a major stigma in Islamic communities. Muslims established psychiatric hospitals as early as 705 CE, and many prominent 11th-century Muslim physicians published important information on the nature of psychiatric disorders. However, Muslims are reluctant to recognize psychiatric illness in their own lives. Often, Muslim patients who have psychiatric problems either are unaware of the problem or attempt to ignore it. They are extremely reluctant to seek psychiatric help, and when they do, they are secretive about it. For health care professionals, it is important to protect the Muslim patient's privacy, especially when discussing psychiatric problems. When approaching these issues, health care providers must also be sensitive to and cognizant of the stigma associated with the topic.

Homosexuality

> We have created everything in pairs. QURAN 51:49

Homosexuality is forbidden in Islamic law. Many Muslims view homosexuality as an illness, a raw, aberrant human desire that must be contained. In the Quran, the practice is condemned as indulged in by the people of Lot, a crime for which they were destroyed. The story recurs in the Quran but is discussed specifically in 11:76. In 7:80, the Quran asserts that the people of Lot committed homosexual acts in an unprecedented manner and scale. The heinousness of homosexual practice is said to consist in the fact that it "obstructs the path" (29:29) of procreation. This teaching poses a major problem for homosexual Muslims, for whom feelings of guilt, disgust, low self-esteem, depression, and isolation are common. The overwhelming majority of gay Muslims either have rejected Islam as their faith or have major emotional and psychological inner conflicts regarding the role of Islam in their lives. Additionally, they are often extremely afraid of persecution.

Fasting, Ramadan, and Medical Treatments

Muslims fast from sunrise to sunset during the holy month of Ramadan. Fasting during Ramadan is regarded as a method of spiritual self-purification, a way of experiencing the suffering of the poor and hungry. The spiritual dimension also involves reflective practices, increased praying, positive thoughts toward other people, and remembrance of God in all thoughts and actions. Muslims consider fasting during Ramadan an important religious duty. Although Muslim jurists have been clear regarding the permissibility of breaking the fast if someone is ill or in need of medical attention, most Muslims (especially ill patients) feel obligated to fast during Ramadan. When Muslim patients who have cancer receive intravenous chemotherapy, for example, they are not able to fast (intravenous therapy technically breaks the Muslim's fast). Muslims greatly appreciate a culturally sensitive physician who is aware when the holy month is observed but also is able to discuss openly with a patient the treatment requirement, whether fasting should be considered an option, and creative ways to allow Muslim patients to fast and continue to be compliant with medical regimens. Typically, any oral medications that are given twice daily can still be continued and taken at different times during Ramadan (at sunrise and at sunset, for example). Generally speaking, Muslim imams in the United States have dealt with these conflicts and are able to provide specific advice to the Muslim patient regarding alternatives to fasting that might be pursued if the patient is very ill or is in dire need of medical treatments during the day.

Genetic Manipulation, Assisted Conception, and Adoption

Quran 95:4, which states that God "created Man in the most perfect form," is often used to explain that each human life has its own inherent value and goodness. Such Islamic principles must not be violated, even when taking into consideration genetic research and the positive impact that gene therapy may have in serving and restoring health. In Islam, an accurate and complete knowledge of one's pedigree is a fundamental human right; therefore, only somatic cell lines should be used in transplantation of genetic material because paternal integrity is then not compromised and there is no question of hereditary characteristics being influenced by others. Children also have the right to be born through a valid union and to know their parentage fully. Artificial insemination and in vitro fertilization are therefore licit only if sperm from the woman's spouse is used.

With regard to adoption, the Prophet stated, "Call the adoptive children by the name of their father." Adoption is generally frowned on in Muslim culture because the legal process in Western countries involves the transfer of parental rights to the adoptive parents. Fostering is encouraged, however, because no similar transfer of parentage occurs. In either case, the surname of the biological father should be retained.

Contraception

Islam has a liberal view on contraception, as is illustrated by the following story: "A man came to the prophet and said, 'We practice coitus interruptus, but we have some Jewish neighbors who say that this is a lesser infanticide.' 'They are lying,' retorted the Prophet. 'It is not lesser infanticide; you may practice it, but if God has predetermined for a child to be born, it will be born" (Rahman 1987, p. 113). The words of Quran 4:3—commonly understood by Muslims to mean "[Marry only one wife], so that you will likely not go wrong"—have been interpreted by Al-Shafii, one of the well-known Muslim jurists, as meaning "So that you will likely not have many children." The overwhelming majority of Muslim theologians and jurists have permitted contraception as long as both the husband and wife agree and are aware of its practice.

Prenatal Screening and Termination of Pregnancy

The Prophet Muhammad wrote, "Each of you will have had his created existence brought together in his mother's womb, as a drop for forty days, then a leech like clot for the same period, then a piece of flesh for the same period, after which God sends the angel to blow the spirit into him" (Sahih Muslim, book 033, Hadith 6390). On the basis of this text, many Muslims conclude that fetal life begins at 120 days after conception (when the soul enters the body). Therefore, first-trimester chorionic villous biopsy and advances in therapeutic fetal medicine are permitted.

Abortion is prohibited, unless it is important to save the mother's life at any point in the pregnancy. It is also allowed in special circumstances of lethal and profound congenital abnormality (preferably within the 120 days after conception).

Child Abuse and Disciplining

> Say: "My Lord, have mercy upon [my parents], as they cared for me in childhood."
>
> QURAN 17:24

The parent-child relationship is considered to be sacred and the most important of all human relationships. Parents and children have mutual rights and responsibilities toward one another, grounded in love, respect, and kindness. Physical, sexual, and emotional abuse of children is thus considered abhorrent and is adamantly rejected by all Muslim jurists within Islamic law. Islamic teaching, however, does allow for parental discipline of children, which may involve physical punishment, but with detailed restrictions. Islamic jurists have agreed that the following conditions must be met: parents must never strike the face or head, minimal force should be used, and no bruising should result from any disciplinary action.

Respecting Patient Autonomy

One important difference between the Islamic view of the physician-patient relationship and the contemporary Western view concerns medical decision making. In contrast to the Western model of informed decision making, in which patients are empowered with the medical information to make the best decision, the Islamic view is that patients should strictly follow their physicians' orders, out of respect, trust, and absolute confidence in their physicians. Muslim patients expect their doctors to carry the burden of decision making because they perceive them as the most knowledgeable. When caring for a Muslim patient, clinicians should describe in detail all the possible therapeutic options but should not be hesitant or resistant to recommending a medical treatment. Often, when the physician takes ownership of the decision, it relieves much of the anxiety and stress that Muslim patients experience in the Western clinical encounter.

In Islam, competent patients have the right to accept or refuse treatment and to be fully informed of their medical condition. This can sometimes be a point of tension, especially when families attempt to protect their loved ones from "bad news" by asking the physician to withhold information. This is a cultural norm with no religious basis. Some Muslim patients appreciate this cultural norm and would rather have their families take full ownership of any clinical decisions to be made, but others feel frustrated and isolated when faced with these difficult situations. In general, the physician taking care of a Muslim patient is often taking care of an entire family. Addressing the needs, worries, and concerns of the family without making general assumptions regarding their values is the first step in cultivating a bond with the patient and the family. A religious leader can often help the clinical team to navigate such challenging cultural dilemmas.

Withholding Life-Sustaining Treatment

Withholding life-sustaining treatment is agreed on by all Muslim jurists and is permissible based on the "Do no harm" principle. For cultural reasons, however, many Muslims believe that they are obligated to do whatever is in their power to treat a life-threatening illness. When families are asked in the medical setting if they would like "everything to be done" for a loved one, they automatically answer "yes." Instead, the discussion should focus on whether the life-sustaining treatments are being used to prolong life with a reasonable hope of recovery or as a means of prolonging the dying process.

According to many Islamic jurists, relentless artificial prolongation of life is ethically appropriate only if there is strong evidence that a reasonable quality of life would result. Muslim jurists have used the "Do no harm" principle in arguing for the permissibility of withdrawing life-sustaining treatment. However, it is important to note that some orthodox Muslim jurists have disagreed with this stance and have forcefully argued the opposite. Specifically, they state, "It is certain that withdrawing treatment will deprive of potential benefits, but uncertain that maintaining will cause harm." When dealing with Muslim families faced with these difficult situations, the clinician should enlist the help of Islamic ethics and legal experts, rather than simply calling on Muslim doctors or imams, who may not posses the appropriate expertise in dealing with these questions. This can be accomplished by first identifying the background of the Muslim family and the specific religious school of thought that they follow, and then consulting with Islamic jurists or medical ethics experts. Health care providers who are informed regarding differences of opinion among Muslim scholars on this subject can often help families navigate within the families' religious network, discuss differing points of view openly, and at times refer families to expert ethicists and scholarly literature written in the field.

Muslim ethicists from the various schools of thoughts are often reachable by the Muslim community, available to answer specific questions that may arise. Trained Muslim imams should be well informed on how to facilitate the communication between the Muslim family and their Islamic school of thought. Trained Muslim imams should also have religious resources, which can be relied on in obtaining the stances of various schools on specific ethical dilemma. It is important to emphasize that the Muslim imam's opinion on the ethical dilemma should not be the guiding force in making a decision. The imam's role should be to educate families regarding the legal and ethical conflicts and how various Muslim scholars have chosen to address them.

Physician-Assisted Suicide and Euthanasia

In Islam, no one is authorized to deliberately end life, whether one's own or that of another human being. Saving life is encouraged. However, alleviating suffering with analgesia is acceptable, even if, in the process, death is hastened. This is based on the central Islamic teaching that "actions are to be judged by their intentions." Withdrawal of food and drink to hasten death is therefore not allowed.

Postmortem Examination and Organ Transplantation

"Breaking the bone of the dead is akin to breaking the bone of the living" (Prophet Muhammad, Sunan Abudawud, book 20, Hadith 3201). This saying underlies the general reluctance of Muslims to allow postmortem examinations. Autopsy is not permitted by most Muslim jurists unless there is a legal requirement to conduct one.

Organ transplantation is an issue that is still open for debate. The majority of Muslim scholars in the Middle East consider it permissible and even encourage it. One of the largest Islamic teaching schools in the Arab world, Al-Azhar, has stated its position on organ transplantation: "If anything was of good for mankind, then the necessity allows what is prohibited under the following conditions: A. the only available treatment is a transplant. B. The likelihood of success is high. C. consent is obtained. D. death of donor has been fully established by a doctor. E. No imminent danger to the life of a living donor" (Gatrad 1994, p. 523).

Addressing and Accessing Spirituality in Practice

Spiritual recitations of the Quran and prayers are at the forefront of traditional Islamic healing rituals. These rituals were approved and conducted by the Prophet Muhammad throughout his life. The Quran is thought to be a "cure" by creating and sustaining faith, and not necessarily by providing a physical cure of illness. According to Al-Dhabai, a famous Muslim traditionalist and historian, the benefits of Islamic ritual prayers are fourfold: spiritual, psychological, physical, and moral:

> Prayers can cause recovery from the pain of the heart, stomach, and intestines. There are three reasons for this.

> First, it is a divinely commanded form of worship.
>
> Second, it has a psychological benefit. This is because prayers divert the mind from the pain and reduce its feeling whereby the power to repel [the cause of] pain is strengthened. Expert doctors try all means to strengthen this [natural] power—sometimes by feeding something, sometimes by inspiring hope, and sometimes by inspiring fear. Now, prayer [with concentration] combines most of these means of benefit, because it at once instills fear, self-effacing humility, love [of God], and remembrance of the Last Day . . . it is related about one of Ali's children that he needed some surgery, but the doctors could not perform it [for fear of causing pain]. His family then left him alone until he embarked on prayers, when they were able to do the surgery—he did not shrink or shrivel because he was deeply concentrating on prayers.
>
> Third, in prayer there is a physical factor (or benefit) as well, besides the concentration of the mind, namely, the exercise of the body. This latter is due to the fact that prayers contain the postures of standing upright, genuflexion, prostration, relaxation, and concentration; where bodily movements occur and most bodily organs relax. . . . Prayers often produce happiness and contentment in the mind; they suppress anxiety and extinguish the fire of anger. They increase love for truth and humility before people; they soften the heart, create love and forgiveness and dislike for the vice of vengeance. Besides, often sound judgment occurs to the mind [due to concentration about difficult matters] and one finds correct answers [to problems]. One also remembers forgotten things . . . one can discover the ways to solve matters worldly and spiritual. And one can effectively examine oneself—particularly when one strenuously exercises oneself in prayers. (Al-Dhahabi, *Prophetic Medicine,* cited in Rahman 1987, p. 44)

In addition to reciting the Quran and prayers, traditional Muslims sometimes use Zamzam's water, which is obtained for its therapeutic properties from the well in the Holy Mosque located in Mecca. The Prophet Muhammad often used honey and black cumin for certain therapeutic remedies. Many Muslims use amulets, but amulets were forbidden by the Prophet.

Although many studies have focused on the role of religious beliefs and values on patients' health care decisions, few have looked at how physicians' cultural and religious values may influence clinical encounters. Yet, 55 percent of physicians agree that their religious beliefs influence their practice of medicine (Curlin et al. 2005). A qualitative study that investigated the perceived influence of Islam on the practice patterns of immigrant Muslim physicians in the United States (Padela et al. 2008) found a great variation in how physicians translated their understanding of Islam into practical action. The authors speculate that this probably stems from physicians' differing cultural, ethnic, educational, and family backgrounds. However, there were some consistent themes: Many physicians felt that virtues taught by an Islamic upbringing upheld the professional ethics of medicine. Physicians also felt that their Islamic background enhanced their work by providing a spiritual dimension to their practice. Islam requires physicians to practice within an exemplary moral realm marked by honesty and accountability to a higher force. To quote one of the Muslim physicians in the study, "Believing that to perfect your work is a form of worship pushes you to do you best in any job you do." Another Muslim physician interviewed stated: "Islam is all about being helpful to others, and medicine is just full of these opportunities to be helpful to mankind and people. If you follow your faith well, it teaches you to be patient, to be just, and to eliminate prejudice." Islam played a role in informing this physician's character development and moral standards.

Some Muslim physicians interviewed by Padela and colleagues perceived Islam as limiting their career choices by defining acceptable medical procedures and shaping their interactions with physician peers. Examples included avoiding obstetrics and gynecology because of the ethical dilemmas associated with abortion, in vitro fertilization, and other reproductive technologies. Some Muslim physicians reported being approached by colleagues to give an "expert opinion" on Islamic-related medical and ethical issues, which they experienced as a burden due to their lack of expertise on these issues.

Muslim physicians identified challenges faced in clinical encounters with patients whose lifestyles were at odds with Islamic teachings (homosexuality was the prominent example given). However, many pointed out the helpfulness of Islamic teachings in being nonjudgmental and treating everyone equally. An additional challenge cited was making decisions regarding withdrawal of medical care at the end of life.

Personal Reflections

Islam has played a tremendous role in shaping my character as a human being and my decision to become a physician. To be an integral part of a profession focusing primarily on giving to others, healing, and alleviating the suffering of patients is a tremendous honor that has become a fundamental aspect of my personal pride. Being a doctor is part of my religion as a Muslim. The amount of joy and pleasure I attain from being a physician is in part due to my religious and spiritual understanding of the sacred importance of this profession. Islam has helped me develop a strong sense of identity, a high moral standard that I am always striving to achieve, and a spiritual satisfaction from practicing the art of medicine. Islam has taught me to be patient, kind, just, and nonjudgmental; to address human suffering physically, emotionally, and mentally; and to create a safe haven for patients.

My spirituality and religion, which are basically one and the same, have empowered me with the ability to discuss spiritual and religious concerns with my patients. I am comfortable approaching the topic with patients, which is often half of the battle. I do not usually disclose my own religious beliefs, but I am capable of asking the right questions. I attempt to gain an understanding of my patients' vision of the world, what sustains them spiritually, mentally, and physically (which may or may not be an organized form of religion). My spiritual background allows me to address the existential suffering that many patients experience when faced with a life-threatening illness.

I believe in prayer and the recital of the Quran as a healing force, and I prescribe it to many of my Muslim patients. This also translates to the care of non-Muslim patients who believe in prayer, meditation, and relaxation techniques. I feel comfortable encouraging patients to pursue any spiritual tools that can bring them comfort and alleviate their suffering.

As a way of life, Islam integrates my life in every dimension, personally and professionally. It provides me with the strength and the ability to surrender to the will of a higher power when in helpless and dire medical situations. It colors my vision of illness, suffering, and the role of a physician in a patient's healing process. Finally and most important, it provides a larger and a more important meaning for my journey in this world by defining my ultimate goals and aspirations.

REFERENCES

Abdul Allah, H. A. 1993. Al-Maliki approach to the Muslim doctrine [in Arabic]. Syria Press.

Ahmed, S. 2005. Tie it and trust. *JAMA* 294:1873–74.

Al-Hilali, M. T., and M. M. Khan. 1994. *Interpretation of the Meanings of the Noble Qur'an in the English Language*. Riyadh, Saudi Arabia: Dar-us-Salam.

Ali, H. A. 2005. Al-Bhukhari: Al-Sharia wal Hayat [in Arabic]. Syria Press.

Ali, S. A. 1983. *The Ethics of Islam*. Calcutta: Thacker Spink.

Al-Jauziyah, I. 1999. *Healing with the Medicine of the Prophet (pbuh)*. Trans. Rab J. Abdul. Riyadh, Saudi Arabia: Dar-us-Salam.

Al-Jibaly, M. 1998. *The Inevitable Journey, Part 1—Sickness: Regulations and Exhortations.* Arlington, TX: Al-Kitaab and As-Sunnah Publishing.

Al-Shahri, M. Z., and A. al-Khenaizan. 2005. Palliative care for Muslim patients. *Journal of Supportive Oncology* 3:432–36.

Beliefnet.com. Faith and Prayer. An Islam Primer. www.beliefnet.com/story/88/story_8830_1.html.

Boobes, Y., and N. Al Daker. 1996. What it means to diet in Islam and modern medicine. *Saudi Journal of Kidney Diseases and Transplantation* 7:121–27.

Brown, D. 2004. *A New Introduction to Islam.* Oxford: Blackwell.

Cheraghi, M. A., S. Payne, and M. Salsali. 2005. Spiritual aspects of end-of-life care for Muslim patients: Experience from Iran. *International Journal of Palliative Nursing* 11:468–74.

Clarfield, A. M., M. Gordon, H. Markwell, and S. M. Alibai. 2003. Ethical issues in end-of-life geriatric care: The approach of three monotheistic religion—Judaism, Catholicism, and Islam. *Journal of the American Geriatrics Society* 51:1149–54.

Curlin, F. A., J. D. Lantos, C. J. Roach, S. A. Sellergren, and M. H. Chin. 2005. Religious characteristics of U.S. physicians: A national survey. *Journal of General Internal Medicine* 20:629–34.

Gatrad, A. R. 1994. Muslim customs surrounding death, bereavement, postmortem examinations, and organ transplants. *British Medical Journal* 309:521–23.

———. 2002. Palliative care for Muslims and issues before death. *International Journal of Palliative Nursing* 8:526–34.

Gatrad, A. R., and A. Sheikh. 2001. Medical ethics and Islam: Principles and practice. *Archives of Disease in Childhood* 84:72–75.

Gibbs, A. R. 1951. *Mohammedanism: An Historical Survey*. London: Oxford University Press.

Goldziher, I. 1981. *Introduction to Islamic Theology and Law*. Princeton, NJ: Princeton University Press.

Hassaballah, A. M. 1996. Definition of death, organ donation and interruption of treatment in Islam. *Nephrology, Dialysis, Transplantation* 11:964–65.

Hedayat, K. 2006. When the spirit leaves: Childhood death, grieving and bereavement in Islam. *Journal of Palliative Medicine* 9:1282–91.

Khan, M. M., trans. 1994. *Summarized Sahih Al-Bukhari*. Riyadh, Saudi Arabia: Dar-us-Salam.

Majlisi, M. B. 1984. *Book 17: Ajr al-Masa'ib, Hadith*. Bihar al-Anwar, Beruit: Mu'assasah al-Wafa 79(4): 115.

Newman, A. J., and I. Batool. 1991. *Islamic Medical Wisdom: The Tibb al-A'imma*. London: Muhammadi Trust.

Ott, B. B., J. Al-Khadhuri, and S. Al-Junaibi. 2003. Preventing ethical dilemmas: Understanding Islamic health care practices. *Pediatric Nursing* 29:227–30.

Padela, A. I., H. Shanawani, J. Greenlaw, H. Hamid, M. Aktas, and N. Chin. 2008. The perceived role of Islam in immigrant Muslim medical practice within the USA: An exploratory qualitative study. *Journal of Medical Ethics* 34:365–69.

Pennachio, D. L. 2005. Caring for your Muslim patients: Stereotypes and misunderstandings affect the care of patients from the Middle East and other parts of the Islamic world. *Medical Economics* 82:46–50.

Pridmore, S., and M. I. Pasha. 2004. Psychiatry and Islam. *Australian Psychiatry* 12:380–85.

Rahman, F. 1979. *Islam*. 2nd ed. Chicago: University of Chicago Press.

———. 1987. *Health and Medicine in the Islamic Tradition: Change and Identity*. New York: Crossroad Publishing.

Rassool, G. H. 2000. The crescent and Islam: Healing, nursing, and the spiritual dimension; Some considerations towards an understanding of the Islamic perspectives on caring. *Journal of Advanced Nursing* 32:1476–84.

Rüschoff, S. I. 1992. The importance of Islamic religious philosophy for psychiatric practice [in German]. *Psychiatrische Praxis* 19(2):39–42.

Sheikh, A. 1998. Death and dying: A Muslim perspective. *Journal of the Royal Society of Medicine* 91:138–40.

Sheikh, A., and A. R. Gatrad. 2000. Death and bereavement: An exploration and a meditation. In *Caring for Muslim Patients*, ed. A. Sheikh and A. R. Gatrad, pp. 97–109. Oxon, UK: Radcliffe Medical Press.

Stein, J. 2006. The bereavement visit in pediatric oncology. *Journal of Clinical Oncology* 24:3705–7.

Shouki, B. 2004. Al- Jaafri and Islamic law [in Arabic]. Syria Press.

Watt, W. M., trans. 1953. *Faith and Practice of Al-Ghazali*. London: Allen & Unwin.

Yasien-Esmael, H., and S. S. Rubin. 2005. The meaning structures of Muslim bereavements in Israel: religious traditions, mourning practices, and human experience. *Death Studies* 29:495–518.

CHAPTER SIX

Christianity

John R. Knight, M.D., and Walter Kim, Ph.D.

Since its inception in the early first century CE, Christianity has become a major global religion. It encompasses a heterogeneous group of cultures, geographical regions, and social strata; adherents now constitute nearly one-third of the world's population. Within this vast network of forms, beliefs, and practices, Christianity is essentially a historical religion centering on the affirmation of God's revelation through Jesus Christ. Its commitment to ethical monotheism entails the belief in a sole deity, who is not an abstract principle or inanimate force. He is a personal being with a mind and volition and a loving and just nature. God interacts generally with the world but has acted most decisively in the historical events surrounding the life, death, and resurrection of Jesus.

Christianity's historical perspective is evident in its sacred scripture, the Bible, which records and interprets God's activity in the world. The Bible demonstrates that Christianity perceives itself as a revealed religion. In addition to divine engagement in history, God discloses or reveals his intentions and desires for the created order. Hence, Christian beliefs and practices flow from the Bible, which comprises two main sections. Christians refer to the Jewish Scriptures as the "Old Testament." These include the five books of Moses and the books of Israelite history, law, poetry, and prophecy. The Christian "New Testament" includes the four gospels (narratives about the life and teachings of Jesus), a book of early church history, a group of letters written by early church leaders, and one book of prophecy.

During the earliest centuries of their experience of God as revealed in Christ, church leaders reached consensus on a statement of faith, known as the Apostles' Creed. Nevertheless, beliefs vary among three major branches: Roman Catholic, Eastern Orthodox, and Protestant subdivisions are known as denominations (Fairchild 2009). Divisions among these groups are for the most part historic and based on differences in theology (i.e., beliefs) and liturgy (i.e., style of worship). Theology varies from liberal to conservative, and liturgy from orthodox to charismatic. Groups also vary in forms of church governance, from hierarchical rule by the clergy (e.g., Catholic, Episcopal) to democratic rule by the local church body (e.g., Congregational).

Beliefs

Although Christians interpret the Bible in various ways, most would agree that certain core beliefs constitute basic Christianity.

1. God intends men and women to be in a harmonious relationship with their creator, with one another, and with the created order.
2. Humankind, both corporately and individually, has broken faith with God's original design. Consequently, we are in a state of "sin" and are thereby condemned to death (Romans 3:23, 6:23).
3. Because of great love for us, God responded by coming in the form of a man, Jesus Christ, and sacrificing his life to pay for the sins of all (John 3:16).
4. If we acknowledge our sins and believe in him, we receive forgiveness and the gift of eternal life.
5. With the resurrection of Jesus, God began a process of restoration in and through the followers of Jesus.

For Christians, moral practice arises as a grateful response to God's activity on behalf of the human predicament. Rather than demonstrating private or abstract virtue, ethical living expresses personal and communal devotion to Christ. In this respect, Christianity is not only a historical and revealed religion but also a relational religion. Belief and devotion revolve around entering into a relationship with God because God has sought out a relationship with humankind through Jesus Christ. According to the Bible, "We love, because God first loved us [in Christ]" (1 John 4:19).

Practices

Religious services vary widely among branches and denominations, but almost all churches assemble weekly on Sunday, which Christians remember as the day of Jesus's resurrection. Some worship services (traditional) are highly stylized, with a set order of hymn singing, scripture reading, group recitations of scripted prayers, and clergy homilies (sermons). Other services (contemporary) may use rock bands, dance, and theatrical presentations to deliver the Christian message. Still others (charismatic) have no set agenda but depend on the "holy spirit" to lead the congregation in spontaneous singing, prayer, teaching, and speaking in "tongues," or prophecies (1 Corinthians 12:7–10). These practices are not mutually exclusive; some churches incorporate diverse elements into worship services.

Christians also practice a variety of rituals, which they call "sacraments." Two—baptism and communion—are recognized by all churches. Baptism with water, which may be accomplished either by anointing the head (children or adults) or by full immersion of the body (adults), is a public acknowledgment of faith in Jesus Christ. Some churches baptize infants on the basis of their parents' faith; others reserve baptism for those who have reached an age of adult understanding and profess their own faith publicly.

Holy Communion, also known as the Eucharist, is a shared symbolic meal. As part of corporate worship, believers mark the last supper that Jesus and his disciples ate together (Luke 22:18–20). Catholic and Orthodox churches distribute wafers or small pieces of bread, which Jesus instructed should represent his body, broken for all. Protestant churches (and some Catholic churches) also distribute wine or grape juice, which Jesus instructed they do as representing his blood, shed for the redemption of sinners everywhere.

Throughout the centuries, Christianity has endeavored to navigate the tension between a uniform commitment to the centrality of Jesus Christ and its pluriform expression. As noted by Huston Smith, a scholar of comparative religions, "From the majestic pontifical High Mass in St. Peter's to the quiet simplicity of a Quaker meeting; from the intellectual sophistication of Saint Thomas

Aquinas to the moving simplicity of spirituals, such as 'Lord, I want to be a Christian'; from St. Paul's in London, the parish church of Great Britain, to Mother Teresa in the slums of Calcutta—all this is Christianity" (Smith 1991, p. 317).

The Ultimate Nature and Essential Concerns of Human Beings

A DOCTOR'S STORY: John R. Knight

The most difficult time of my professional life occurred in my mid-30s. I had graduated from an excellent college and a great medical school, but I did not complete the third year of my residency. Instead, I entered the new field of emergency medicine. I thought the excitement, limited hours, and financial rewards would make me happy. However, I found nothing that could fill a growing emptiness inside me. I lost interest in my career, family, and everything else I had once loved; and I descended into a state of emotional pain and spiritual darkness. One day, out of complete desperation, I prayed to a God whom I wasn't sure even existed: "God, I offer myself to you, to do with me and to build with me as you will. Relieve me of the bondage of self, that I may better do your will. Take away my difficulties, that my victory over them may bear witness to those I would help of your power, your love, and your way of life. May I do your will always." Through the years that followed, I discovered that God does indeed exist and that he does answer prayer.

Why Are We Here?

According to the Westminster Catechism, the chief end of mankind "is to glorify God and to enjoy him forever" (Williamson 2003). Glorifying God begins with believing in him; we then can delight in his daily presence in our lives. For the Christian, coming to faith is not merely intellectual assent to a creed but a vibrant personal relationship with God. It begins with a simple prayer. We confess that we are sinners, ask for forgiveness, and ask God to take over our lives and to use us for his purpose (Romans 10:9). The prayer is simple but not necessarily easy. We must completely surrender our lives and wills to the care of God. This is a spiritual paradox: only through surrender can we achieve victory.

Christians believe that people are sinners from the moment of conception (Psalm 51:5). This means not that humans are evil but that we are imperfect.

Despite our unworthiness, God, in his infinite love and mercy, unconditionally elects us to receive his salvation (Romans 8:29–30). We need only have faith in order to receive it (Ephesians 2:8). God then applies his irresistible grace to our lives, which draws us inexorably toward him. "Grace" is a free and unmerited gift from God (Ephesians 2:8). We choose only whether we will receive it. Christians cannot earn salvation through righteous living or good deeds. Jesus taught that we must love and serve all and dedicate everything we have to advancing his kingdom. However, these "good works" do not redeem us; they are merely a means of showing gratitude for the gift God has freely bestowed on us.

A DOCTOR'S STORY (CONTINUED)

Just a few years after coming to faith, I went on a job search. One possibility, at the top of my list, was to become director of urgent care for a large physician-owned group practice, a job which offered a pleasant lifestyle and generous financial package. Out of curiosity only, I also visited a state school for individuals with developmental disabilities that was advertising for a primary care physician. Just before I signed a contract for the urgent care position, the state school's medical director asked me to meet with him a second time. I reluctantly agreed. He then shared with me his own journey of faith. After completing residency, he turned down a staff position at a nationally known teaching hospital to become a medical missionary in Haiti. After 11 years, medical problems forced him to return to the United States, where he became director of emergency services at another prominent hospital. One day, he accompanied a friend on a visit to the state school. When he saw helpless, restrained patients, lying in their own waste, God touched his heart and told him, "This is your new mission field."

I listened to his story politely, thanked him, and left feeling troubled. I prayed, "Oh, no, Lord, surely you don't expect me to work there?" Well, God was testing me. Did I really mean it when I offered my life to him? Was I really willing to do his will? After a night of painful soul searching, I accepted the position at the state school. It turned out to be a wonderful experience. It took me down a career path I could never have imagined, and ultimately led to my current faculty appointment and hospital position at Harvard Medical School/Children's Hospital Boston.

The story of the two thieves crucified with Jesus is a noteworthy example of the simplicity of coming to faith. One thief mocked Jesus. The other rebuked the first, saying, "We are punished justly, for we are getting what our deeds deserve. But this man has done nothing wrong." Then he turned to Jesus and said, "Lord, remember me when you come into your kingdom." Jesus replied, "I tell you the truth, today you will be with me in paradise" (Luke 23: 41–43).

Glorifying God

The simplest and most direct ways of glorifying God are through praise, songs, and prayers of thanksgiving (Psalm 69:30). We can also glorify God by telling others of his great love for us, by acknowledging him as the reason for our achievements and by maintaining our faith during hardships. Immediately after one of his disciples betrayed him and set in motion events that would lead to his death, Jesus stated, "Now is the Son of Man glorified and God is glorified in him." Many of Jesus's followers viewed him as the promised Messiah king, who would free them from Roman oppression and reestablish the Jewish nation. Yet Jesus announced to them that it would be through his death that God would receive true glory. In similar fashion, we can glorify God by trusting and praising him during difficult times.

Enjoying God

The experience of God's love, the gift of salvation, and the promise of transformation all contribute to what the Bible describes and Christians experience as being "filled with an inexpressible and glorious joy" (1 Peter 1:8). When we surrender all we are and all we have to him, God fills our emptiness with his peace, freedom, and joy. He relieves us of the bondage of self-centered desire and replaces it with the joy of giving to others. Joy also comes through the many blessings we receive: friendships, family, children, pets, delicious foods, bright sunny days, breathtaking landscapes, and all the other wonders of creation. Thus, communion with God is the essential foundation for discovering what it means to be truly human.

Suffering and Death

Rabbi Harold Kushner, in his landmark book, *When Bad Things Happen to Good People*, describes the pain of watching his son die from progeria (Kushner 2004). Kushner cannot reconcile the suffering of an innocent child with a God who is both all-powerful and all-loving. However, this dissonance exists only if we consider life on earth to be all we have. If, instead, our human experience is only a small part of eternal existence, which we will spend in God's presence, then "our present sufferings are not worth comparing with the glory that will be revealed in us" in the new life to come (Romans 8:18).

Suffering makes a Christian grow, not because it is good, but because we must draw closer to God during trials, and he assures us he will provide the means for us to endure. God also promises that he will cause all things to work together for our good, if we love him, follow his calling, and fulfill his purpose for our lives (Romans 8:28). Furthermore, Christians approach the issue of suffering with the knowledge of how God himself, in human form, suffered for us on the cross. Christians are not exempt from death or from sadness, but we have the promise of eternal life after death. The Apostle Paul therefore boldly asks, "Where, O death, is your victory? Where, O death, is your sting?" (Philippians 1:21).

Resurrection

Christian faith depends on believing in a physical resurrection; it is otherwise nothing more than a philosophy of right thinking and good deeds. However, for a physician, no single tenet of Christianity may be harder to accept. Doctors have the sad misfortune of observing many deaths and never witnessing anyone coming back to life. They also learn of the complexities of brain structure and chemistry, how quickly lack of oxygen disrupts them, and that the ensuing brain death is irreversible. How then could anyone ever return from the dead?

Faith in life eternal begins with belief in Jesus's resurrection. Some charge that his disciples concocted this story. Such a contrivance makes little sense. First, there is the evidence of his empty tomb. There was no debate at the time that his body was missing. If his disciples invented this story, others would have refuted it by simply bringing out Jesus's body. Then there is the self-evident lie of the Roman guards: "His disciples came during the night and stole him away while we were asleep" (Matthew 28:13). How could they possibly know what happened while they were sleeping? Next, no thinking person of that time would invent a story in which the first witnesses to discover the empty tomb were women. In Jesus's day, many regarded women as too unreliable to testify in court. It would have been much simpler to invent a story in which the first witnesses were prominent men. Last, all but one of Jesus's disciples were eventually put to death for their beliefs. While many will die for a truth, few are willing to die for their own lie. Nonetheless, in the final analysis, belief in Jesus's resurrection is a matter of faith. Without faith, it is impossible to please God, because anyone who comes to him must believe that he exists and that he rewards those who seek him (Hebrews 11:6).

A DOCTOR'S STORY (CONTINUED)

After seven years of attending regularly, I decided to join my church. Toward the end of a series of membership classes, the teacher asked us to sign a "Statement of Faith." My heart sank when I read it. Like the Apostles' Creed, it included a statement about belief in the resurrection. My faith was too weak to sign it, so I dropped out of the class. For years after that, I felt like a second-class Christian, especially on those Sundays when I watched other people welcomed into church membership. I met with one of the ministers to discuss this. He pointed me to a story in Mark 9 about a man who came to Jesus seeking healing for his son. Jesus said to him, "Everything is possible for him who believes." The man exclaimed, "I do believe; help me overcome my unbelief!" I had read this story before but had never noticed the contradiction. The minister explained that faith is not unidimensional; it has a component of strength. This struck an immediate chord with me. I had been looking at faith as a dichotomous variable, when in fact it is a continuous one. I was able to make peace with my own weakness, knowing that God loves us so much, he accepts us just as we are. A few months later, I became a member of the church.

Injustice

Because justice is part of the character of God and the mission of Christ, Christians must seek justice on behalf of others. Jesus taught us to turn the other cheek but never to turn our backs. Outrage at injustice is a way of showing love to the downtrodden, the oppressed, and the wronged. The Book of Esther provides a powerful story about speaking out for the powerless. Esther is a Jewish girl who becomes queen of Persia at a time when the king issues a proclamation of genocide against all Jews. Esther's uncle pleads with her to intervene with the king on behalf of her people. Esther initially refuses, saying that anyone who enters the king's presence uninvited is immediately put to death. Her uncle responds, "If you remain silent at this time, relief and deliverance for the Jews will arise from another place, but you and your father's family will perish. And who knows but that you have come to royal position for such a time as this?" (Esther 4:14).

A DOCTOR'S STORY (CONTINUED)

For 15 years I held a consulting position with a state not-for-profit organization whose mission was to help individuals with mental health problems. This work was meaningful to me as a Christian believer, but it also provided an important financial supplement to my academic salary. Over the course of those years, I became concerned about a drift I perceived in the philosophy of the program, from one that was about helping clients to another that was more administrative and punitive. Finally, it became painfully clear to me that I could not continue to work for the organization unless its leaders were willing to make changes. I was still reluctant to speak up, but one Sunday the annual performance by the children's choir presented the story of Queen Esther, and I knew God was speaking to my heart.

Most Christian doctors live privileged lives. I certainly do. Who knows but that God gives us prestigious titles and appointments, incomes well above average, and the respect and admiration of the public, all so that we can be in a better position to speak up for the downtrodden and powerless? I spoke up and lost my position, and have no regrets. I thank God for considering me worthy to make this small sacrifice for the sake of his kingdom.

Insights about Life and Healing

Well-Being

Jesus demonstrated a profound concern for the well-being of those who were physically infirm. Although the Bible does not use contemporary psychological language, it displays an equal concern for our emotional health. Christianity therefore affirms the work of modern medicine to promote physical and psychological wellness. God designed his law for our well-being, but our persistent tendency to live apart from God burdens us and keeps us from experiencing the full blessing of his plan for us. This does not mean that every sickness results from shortcomings. It does mean that our well-being flows from the restoration of healthy relationships with God, one another, and creation.

Peace of Mind

Many of us carry heavy burdens that we have placed on ourselves. For doctors, these include working long hours far beyond their job descriptions and constantly dealing with human pain, illness, and death. Those in academic medicine carry additional burdens, such as constant pressure to secure grant funding, publish, and achieve tenure and promotion. Like Marley's ghost, we wear the chains that we forge for ourselves, link by link, and we wear them of our own free will (Dickens 1843, chap. 1, p. 24). Jesus said, "Come to me, all you who are weary and burdened, and I will give you rest. Take my yoke upon you and learn from me, for I am gentle and humble in heart, and you will find rest for your souls. For my yoke is easy and my burden is light" (Matthew 11:28–30).

Reinhold Niebuhr's "Serenity Prayer," adopted by Alcoholics Anonymous, summarizes how Christian faith can help us find peace of mind even in the midst of great turmoil. For some of us, spiritual serenity may be the only viable alternative to self-medication with alcohol and other psychoactive substances.

Healing

Jesus healed many people. He often accompanied the healing by forgiving sins and citing the importance of faith (Acts 3:16). This leads some to believe in "faith healing," a doctrine that proclaims that you will be healed if your faith is strong enough. If this were true, many Christians would never die. In fact, all who have preceded us, including the founders of the ancient church, have died. Some were martyred, but most died from ordinary human ailments. Faith healing impugns these men and women by implying that their faith was insufficient. This is a particularly cruel implication for Christian believers near the end of life.

Faith healing is part of a "health and wealth" gospel, often preached via television. Its basic tenet is that Christians are the chosen children of God and as such are entitled to perfect health and great wealth. It is true that God has chosen us to be his children. However, he does not promise us freedom from poverty or illness, but only to help us endure them. In fact, he calls many of us to lives of self-sacrifice. Jesus taught his disciples, "If anyone would come after me, he must deny himself and take up his cross and follow me" (Matthew 16:24).

Divine healing, by contrast, flows from the belief that God can heal anyone, but that he chooses whom he will heal according to his own purposes. When God chooses not to heal us, he is still manifesting his grace in our lives. Helping us to endure suffering, even death, provides evidence to those around us of the power of God to strengthen and sustain us. Divine healing is uncommon, which is why we refer to it as a miracle. The Apostle Paul wrote of receiving a "thorn in the flesh" as a way of keeping him humble. We do not know the exact nature of his malady, but it clearly was distressing. Three times, he asked God to heal him, but that did not happen. Instead, God responded to his request, "My grace is sufficient for you, for my power is made perfect in weakness" (2 Corinthians 12:9).

Christian doctors are not exempt from suffering. However, God promises that his grace will be with us in times of need (Hebrews 4:16). Furthermore, he charges us to walk through life helping others as an expression of his plan for humankind to live harmoniously in community. However, a vocation of service requires the enabling of God's strength. The Bible uses an agricultural metaphor to explain virtue: "The fruit of the Spirit is love, joy, peace, patience, kindness, goodness, faithfulness, gentleness, and self-control" (Galatians 5:22–23). A prayer attributed to St. Francis of Assisi is a good description of the Christian's duty to help others and of our need for divine assistance in order to be successful.

Relationship to Contemporary Medical Practice

The practice of medicine today involves many conflicts and controversies. Doctors must balance the quality of care with the economic necessity of treating more patients more quickly. At a policy level, we must all balance the need to control the continually rising costs of health care with the expense of providing the best care to the sick and disabled. Abortion and end-of-life decisions are steeped in a swirl of competing moral principles that force even the most sincere and discerning Christians to proceed with caution. Beyond these specific issues, there remain the philosophical presuppositions of contemporary medicine, which may sometimes be at variance with a Christian worldview. Nonetheless, interaction between medicine and faith presents numerous opportunities for mutual benefit. Medicine's commitment to beneficence and service to humanity coincides with fundamental aspirations of Christians. For this reason, medicine has always been an attractive field for practicing believers.

As is often the case with matters of profound complexity and importance, the biggest struggle resides at the most rudimentary level of conflicting worldviews. The belief in human accountability to God results in a particular evaluation of human value and dignity and of our calling to lay down our lives for one another and to trust God during times of suffering. In contrast, a worldview that is grounded in secular humanism yields a different set of values and agendas, such as the right to choose and control one's own destiny.

Abortion

One author of this chapter is the father of two adopted children. He thanks God for the courage of their birth mothers, who chose to give them life in the midst of personal crises, and he prays that God will richly reward them for giving his wife and him the priceless gift of family. The other author is the father of a beautiful girl who happens to have Down syndrome. He prays that other expectant parents who receive this diagnosis prenatally will choose the joys of parenthood and family over terminating the pregnancy.

Nonetheless, we believe it our duty as Christians to love and support women facing crisis pregnancies, regardless of their decisions. A small but visible minority of Christians protest outside women's health centers, shouting at those going in, "Don't murder your child," while holding up photos of aborted fetuses. If Jesus were on earth today, we believe he would not participate in these activities. However, we can see him standing quietly by the clinic door, offering help and support to those going in as well as unconditional love and healing to those coming out. We believe in working to make most abortions unnecessary, by providing tangible supports to women in crisis. We also believe in reaching out in love to those who suffer from abortion's aftereffects.

A DOCTOR'S STORY (CONTINUED)

During a recent service at my church, I witnessed a special service of baptism for a six-month-old baby. Her father told us the story of how his young wife, stricken with a particularly aggressive form of cancer during her pregnancy, had chosen to forgo chemotherapy and not have an abortion, thereby sacrificing her own life so that her unborn child might have a chance to live. The chances that she would carry this baby to term and have a live birth were poor; the chances of her baby's having a normal life, without severe disabilities, were even poorer. Yet, on this day, I saw a beautiful, bright-eyed, developmentally normal little girl, babbling in her father's arms. He told us that his wife had only a few brief moments to see her newborn child in the NICU; she lost her battle with cancer a few days after giving birth. He described how God sustained him through the struggle with depression that followed losing the love of his life.

While the minister baptized this tiny miracle in the name of the Father, Son, and Holy Spirit, her four-year old sister cavorted happily across the platform behind her daddy. He gazed lovingly at the baby in his arms; she looked up into his proud and happy face. How conflicted I felt: sad for his loss, amazed by his resilience, awed by the joy of this family who would be forever incomplete, and inspired by this story of how the sacrificial love of Christ and simple faith of a young couple had wrought something so incredibly beautiful.

End of Life

As Christians, we take issue with those supporting "assisted suicide" over appropriate and compassionate end-of-life care. God provides his grace during times of need, and the dying are not exceptions. Medical science offers many effective options for treatment of pain, depression, and anxiety. We deplore the withholding or minimal dosing of narcotic analgesics for those who have malignant pain. We firmly believe that the medical profession should focus its efforts on better systems of care for the chronically ill and dying (e.g., hospice care) and not become a party to the delivery of death. Hippocrates understood the importance of keeping physicians as guardians of life. The oath that bears his name states: "I will prescribe regimens for the good of my patients according to my ability and my judgment and never do harm to anyone. I will not give a lethal drug to anyone if I am asked, nor will I advise such a plan."

How Beliefs Influence Practice

A DOCTOR'S STORY (CONTINUED)

After I had worked at the state school for individuals with developmental disabilities for about a year, the state cut the medical services contract budget. The director had no choice but to let one physician go. He chose a part-time person, who threatened to file a grievance with the state labor board unless he let me go instead. I was incredulous as I sat in his office and he told me that I would have to leave. Later, I prayed, "Lord, how can you let this happen? I sacrificed a better job opportunity to accept this one. I was trying to do your will." I was confused, hurt, and angry. The director told me not to worry. God had something else for me to do.

Over the next few days, after another painful round of soul searching, I saw that God was testing me again. This time it was a matter of faith. Did I really believe that God had a plan for my life, that he would make all things work together for my good? I prayed for stronger faith. I prayed for a new job. I also prayed for the doctor who demanded that I be let go. I continued to be friendly to her. The medical services contract was through a major university hospital. When leaders there heard what had happened, that I maintained a positive attitude and was not angry with the other doctor, they offered me a much better position. This was a dream come true for me. I have been at that hospital now for more than 20 years.

Several other times during my career, people have treated my unkindly, tried to use or abuse me, blamed me for something unjustly, or otherwise betrayed my friendship. My duty as a Christian was to forgive them, to pray for them, and to love them unconditionally, as God loves me. Each time, my career has advanced to a new and better direction.

Forgiveness

We must seek forgiveness for our own moral failures and freely grant forgiveness to others for theirs, even if they never ask us to forgive them. Christians refer to moral failure as "sin." In the original biblical languages, this word could be used to tell archers they had missed the mark, and so has a figurative meaning of "missing a moral standard." The scripture is clear on this issue: all have sinned and fallen short of the glory of God (Romans 3:23). Forgiveness of others is not an option for Christians; it is a requirement. Jesus told a parable about two servants, one of whom owed his master a huge amount of money, which the master forgave. This servant then turned around and demanded repayment from a fellow servant who owed him a substantial amount (a few months' salary), but a tiny fraction of his own forgiven debt. When the master heard of this, he reversed his decision to forgive the massive debt and turned the unforgiving servant over to jailers to be tortured until he repaid his entire original debt. "This is how my heavenly Father will treat each of you unless you forgive your brother from your heart" (Matthew 18:21–35). The duty of the injured is to forgive. However, the duty of those around the injured is to comfort and protect them and to seek justice on their behalf (Knight and Hugenberger 2007).

Love All, Serve All

As a religion that centers on Jesus, Christianity considers him to be the embodiment of the ideal and the good. Consequently, the ideal takes the form of a person rather than a principle. The ideal flows from what he teaches, what he exemplifies, and what he produces. At one point Jesus was asked, "Teacher, which is the greatest commandment in the Law?" Jesus replied: "Love the Lord your God with all your heart and with all your soul and with all your mind. This is the first and greatest commandment. And the second is like it: 'Love your neighbor as yourself.' All the Law and the Prophets hang on these two commandments" (Matthew 22:36–40).

In the effort to live out these fundamental commands, Christians have traditionally pursued the "imitation of Christ" as a primary rubric of spirituality. His injunctions become our pursuits: love everyone (John 13:34–35) including your enemies (Matthew 5:44), serve all humankind, feed the hungry, clothe the naked, visit the prisoner, and heal the sick. "Whatever you did for one of the least of these brothers of mine, you did for me" (Matthew 25:34–40). His example of ministering to the outcasts and downtrodden of his day, and ultimately his crucifixion, serve as our models of service and self-sacrifice. Christians also have a realistic view of human nature as dichotomous, with potential for both good and evil. For this reason, Christians recognize the inadequacy of human efforts alone to achieve the ideal, and the good. Christian character requires the transformative work of God's Spirit in the individual and in society.

A DOCTOR'S STORY (CONTINUED)

Halfway through my academic career, I was the acting chief on one of the hospital's three inpatient medical services. I loved this role. The department was planning to switch over to a hospitalist system, and I wanted to be part of it. But something happened. A teenager whom I had watched grow up in my neighborhood, the only son of a physician colleague who lived in a house behind ours, disappeared from the edge of an abandoned granite quarry where he and a few friends had gone to drink. Divers recovered his body four hours later. The 6 o'clock news showed his father climbing into the back of a rescue truck to identify his only son's body. I could not get that image out of my mind. But for the grace of God, that could have been my son, anyone's son. God was calling me to a new mission field.

As a world-class teaching hospital, we had a program for every disease known to mankind but one: substance abuse. I changed my career direction in response. I began a small clinic, the Adolescent Substance Abuse Program, which was the first of its kind to be located at a children's hospital in the United States. This year our staff of almost 20 will accommodate more than 3,000 visits. God also used me to establish a research center that develops and tests new strategies for pediatric office management of substance abuse. Our screening and brief intervention strategies are now used across the United States and in a growing number of foreign countries, saving many young lives and futures. I love what I do and what God is doing through me.

Spirituality in Practice

A DOCTOR'S STORY (CONTINUED)

I pray for patients all the time, but in private. I sometimes ask, "Is it OK if I add you to my prayer list?" as a way of showing that I care. No one has ever said no. I do not ask patients if I can pray with them during the medical visit. Patients who depend on me for their care might agree only because they don't wish to offend me. I never proselytize at work. However, co-workers and trainees often seek me out to ask for advice. I cannot explain how I make career decisions without mentioning my faith. However, I first ask permission, "Would it be OK for me to tell you how my religious beliefs influenced me in a similar situation?" No one has ever said no. A coworker, who is also a Christian, once asked if we could start an early morning Bible study in our conference room. I told him that he could, but that I would not be able to attend. Because I am the director, my participation might make non-Christians uncomfortable, even create a subtle climate of coercion. It is better for me to read my Bible and pray in privacy.

The high regard that our society has for physicians gives them great influence in patient encounters. Doctors must never take advantage of their power for personal reasons. The doctor-patient relationship must be based on patient autonomy, trust, and mutual respect. It is therefore improper for doctors to proselytize for their own religion in doctor-patient encounters or to ask patients to join them in religious behaviors in which they would not otherwise engage.

The Spiritual History

There is a growing body of evidence on the beneficial effects of spirituality on health, even among children (Knight et al. 2007; Chida, Steptoe, and Powell

2009). Patients who have a serious illness or chronic disorder may benefit from spiritual support and counseling. It is therefore appropriate for doctors to ask about religion and spirituality as a standard part of their usual psychosocial assessment. Two questions can efficiently open this discussion: "What is your religious or spiritual worldview?" and "How can I help provide for your spiritual needs?" When seeing patients in a hospital or other health care facility, the clinician may find it appropriate to ask if the patient would like to speak with a chaplain and, if so, from what religion.

Prayer

Praying for patients is not the same as praying with patients. We believe it is always appropriate to pray for patients, during a private prayer time outside of the medical encounter. Jesus instructed his followers to pray in secret, perhaps to avoid the temptation of seeking attention through public display: "But when you pray, go into your room, close the door and pray to your Father, who is unseen. Then your Father, who sees what is done in secret, will reward you" (Matthew 6:6). Some patients may respond to the question about helping to meet spiritual needs by asking that a doctor pray for them. Few patients will ask a doctor to pray with them. If one does, there is no reason to refuse. In fact, it is a powerful way to express caring and concern. However, asking a patient if you can pray with them should be reserved for those whom you know are fellow Christian believers.

The same principles hold true for doctors who are medical school faculty, hospital chiefs, or otherwise in a position of power over students, trainees, other physicians, or hospital or laboratory staff. They should not use their positions to proselytize or suggest that others join them in religious practices unless they have prior knowledge that the individual shares their religious faith. This does not mean that we cannot remember them in our usual prayer time. To the contrary, we should pray that God would show us ways to bless them daily through our words and deeds. It is by unconditional love and service to those around us that we have the greatest opportunity to spread the good news of the Gospel.

Humility

One of the most powerful examples of humble service took place at the last supper. Jesus removed his outer rabbinical garments and donned a servant's garb. He took a water-filled basin and a cloth, kneeled before each disciple, and one by one, washed their feet. Presumably, this also included Judas, the disciple who within minutes would betray him. Thus, the one whom we regard as the Son of God willingly became the servant. He then instructs us: "Now that I, your Lord and Teacher, have washed your feet, you also should wash one another's feet" (John 13:1–17).

For Christians, all genuine service is a reflection of Christ's ultimate expression of love, when he laid down his life on a cross. We must be willing to embrace personal sacrifice in order to lift others up. However, Christians believe that Jesus's death is not only a model for us to emulate, but also the means by which our lives transform, making such an imitation possible. In the forgiveness of sins and the liberation from self-centeredness that takes place at the cross, Christians discover the freedom and joy required to follow Christ's example.

A DOCTOR'S STORY (CONCLUDED)

When it comes to sharing my faith, I believe that Christianity is better suited to a demonstration than a lecture. I pray each day that God will help me love people unconditionally and serve them without any thought of thanks or reward. It is best to do good deeds secretly. I also ask for a spirit of humility. Doctors often hold the power of life and death over others. If we aren't careful, we can start to believe we are gods. As a Christian, I strive to emulate Jesus's example of humility and service in all I do. One of my favorite scripture passages is Philippians 2:5–8: "Your attitude should be the same as that of Christ Jesus: Who, being in very nature God, did not consider equality with God something to be grasped, but made himself nothing, taking the very nature of a servant, being made in human likeness. And being found in appearance as a man, he humbled himself and became obedient to death—even death on a cross!" Of course, I often fail in my Christian walk. No one should be surprised when that happens. Rather, people should be surprised when I achieve something great. I am nothing more than a weak and foolish believer struggling daily to live out my faith. I ask for God's power to flow through my weaknesses and to be "foolish" enough to risk everything I have to accomplish his will.

REFERENCES

Chida, Y., A. Steptoe, and L. H. Powell. 2009. Religiosity/spirituality and mortality: A systematic quantitative review. *Psychotherapy and Psychosomatics* 78:81–90.

Dickens, C. 1843. *A Christmas Carol.* Electronic Text Center, University of Virginia Library. http://etext.lib.virginia.edu/modeng/modengD.browse.html. Accessed 11 Nov. 2009.

Fairchild, M. Christianity Today: General Statistics and Facts of Christianity. http://christianity.about.com/od/denominations/p/christiantoday.htm. Accessed 19 Nov. 2009.

Knight, J. R., and G. P. Hugenberger. 2007. On forgiveness. *Southern Medical Journal* 100:420–21.

Knight, J. R., L. Sherritt, S. K. Harris, et al. 2007. Alcohol use and religiousness/spirituality among adolescents. *Southern Medical Journal* 100:349–55.

Kushner, H. 2004. *When Bad Things Happen to Good People.* New York: Anchor Books.

Smith, H. C. 1991. *The World's Religions: Our Great Wisdom Traditions.* New York: HarperCollins.

Williamson, G. I. 2003. *The Westminster Shorter Catechism: For Study Classes.* 2nd ed. Phillipsburg, NJ: P & R Publishing.

CHAPTER SEVEN

Buddhism

Robert Wall, M.Div., M.S.N., F.N.P.-B.C., A.P.M.H.N.P.-B.C.

A Buddhist responds to illness, change, and death with an integrated philosophy and practice that is instructive to care providers in all healing traditions. The best way to understand a Buddhist is to gain an appreciation of how Buddhists practice mindfulness and compassion. Insight meditation, Zen meditation, mindfulness-based stress reduction (see the appendix to this chapter), and Tibetan Vajrayana are a few of the choices available in the West today. In this chapter, I offer some background for such a quest, by considering who the Buddha was and what he taught, what research into mindfulness has shown, and how these teachings function in approaching life, suffering, and the end of life.

The Ultimate Nature and Essential Concerns of Human Beings

Buddhism began with a man born Siddhartha Gautama of the Sakya tribal republic living in a part of India that is now Nepal, in 563 BCE. He left his home, and after six years of arduous spiritual practice he attained enlightenment. He was called by his followers "The Buddha"; the title means "one who knows" or "one who is awake." Its root, *budh*, comes into the English language as a verb "to bud (forth)," in the sense of a tree or flower budding or blooming, and by extension ourselves, when we awaken. When asked if he was a god, the Buddha replied, "No, I am not a god. I am awake." Being awake in Buddhist parlance is not the opposite of being asleep. It contrasts with "forgetting" the present moment and by implication forgetting who you are. The Buddha's story asks everyone, "Who and what are you?" and his story provides the answer: "I am awake" (Smith and Novak 2003, p. 4).

The Buddha taught for 45 years until he died at 80 years of age, in 483 BCE. What is left to us are the basic teachings he named the Four Noble Truths and the Eightfold Path. In modern terms, the Truths and the Path are a program of instruction whose thesis is that suffering can be ended, or significantly reduced, through rigorous and systematic cognitive-behavioral practices based in mindfulness. The Four Noble Truths express four objectives: (1) to name suffering; (2) to name what causes it; (3) to name what can be done to end it; and (4) to prescribe the way to end it.

The first insight, or Truth, is the importance of naming suffering. Huston Smith and Philip Novak, in their superb primer *Buddhism*, observe that suffering arises from our resistance to the superficiality and boredom of mundane life, which leaves "deep regions of the human psyche empty and wanting." The Buddha called this deep objective dissatisfaction *dukkha*. The word has an onomatopoetic component, deriving from the sound a cart makes when its wheel is attached to a bent axle—dukkha-dukkha-dukka. It is an irritating "sound" that life makes when it does not go the way we want or expect. Human life is marked by dukkha, and the following events are inescapable:

- the trauma of birth
- sickness
- fear of morbidity
- fear of death
- being tied to what one dislikes
- separation from what and whom one loves

Jon Kabat-Zinn remarked in his book *Full Catastrophe Living* that he found this title in Nikos Kazantsakis's novel *Zorba the Greek*. Zorba answered an inquiry as to whether he was married or not: "Of course, I'm married. I have a wife, children, the full catastrophe!" (Kabat-Zinn 1990, p. 5). The full catastrophe is a good metaphor for what the Buddha meant by impermanence and is used here to stand in for all that impermanence means.

The second insight, or Truth, involves naming what causes suffering: our conditioned expectation and fixed ideas that life will be permanent and unchanging. Suffering occurs when we resist life's unsatisfactoriness, when we rail against impermanence (the constant state of flux, or *anitya*), disbelieve our interdependence on all other things (nonself, or *anatman*), and attempt to evade the full catastrophe. The ancient Sanskrit word for the "desire that resists" is *tanha*, meaning a selfish craving to avoid suffering, change, and unpleasantness while accruing power, admiration, and pleasure for oneself. I find helpful an algorithm offered by Shinzen Young (2009) to encapsulate this: $S = P \times R$ (i.e., suffering equals pain times resistance). Resistance to pain exponentially drives up suffering. Practicing various attentional skills that engender equanimity or nonreactivity has been shown to decrease the perception of pain by inducing what has been called "acceptance and nonstriving," which taps the body's power to heal and resiliency (Kabat-Zinn 1990, p. 89; Mollica 2006; Williams et al. 2007, p. 67).

The third insight, or Truth, involves naming what can be done about suffering: learning and practicing the skills that decrease resistance and self-centered craving. Those skills are embedded within the cognitive-behavioral approach that is known as the fourth insight, or Truth. In Buddhist parlance, this fourth Truth is called the Noble Eightfold Path, or, as I suggest, living the full catastrophe (Nhat Hanh 1998):

Wisdom
1. Right view
2. Right intention

Ethical conduct
3. Right speech
4. Right action
5. Right occupation
6. Right effort

Mental development
7. Right mindfulness
8. Right concentration

Exploring any one step will lead in a circular way to the others. These eight steps are similar to other ethical guides—for example, the twelve steps of Alcoholics Anonymous. Just as the twelve steps, though rooted in the U.S. Christian tradition, provide a way of living a nonaddictive, ethical life without necessarily making one a Christian, the eight steps of the Buddhist cultural tradition provide a cognitive-behavioral method of ethical living that makes one, not necessarily a Buddhist, but rather, more fully human (Nhat Hanh 1996).

The details of the Eightfold Path are beyond the scope of this chapter but are available in several good works on the Buddha's teaching (Nhat Hanh 1998; Smith and Novak 2003; Weiss 2004). Several scholars (Batchelor 1994; Coleman 2000; Maezumi and Glassman 2002; Smith and Novak 2003) have written eminently readable accounts of how Buddhist practice and mindfulness came into U.S. and other Western cultures.

Three major tributaries, differing in their emphasis owing to their country of origin, contribute to Buddhist practice in the West. The Mahayana form (practiced in Japan, China, Korea, and Vietnam) is associated with Zen and the Pure Land tradition (Nhat Hanh 1996). The other two forms are Tibetan Vajrayana Buddhism (from Tibet, Nepal, and India) and Theravadan Vipassana Buddhism (practiced in Burma/ Myanmar, Thailand, Vietnam, and Cambodia). Vipassana Buddhism (*vipassana is* Sanskrit for "insight") is most often associated with the practice of mindfulness (Goldstein and Kornfield 1987; Smith and Novak 2003).

Zen connotes to most Americans a refined, calm Asian style in clothing, gardening sensibility, and furniture. *Zen* in Japanese means "to sit," and *za* means "stillness"; hence, *zazen* means "to sit still." *Zen* is originally a translation of the Chinese word *C'han,* describing the rigorous sitting meditation method of Buddhism. In Korea it is *Son*, and in Vietnam *Thien*. Zen came to Western shores originally during the early and middle 20th century from Japan's two Zen schools, Soto and Rinzai Zen.

Zen meditation, Tibetan Vajrayana practices, and Vipassana Insight meditation all develop concentration, which in turn produces mindfulness. The mindfulness component of the Eightfold Path has been the most rigorously studied for its clinical utility (Baer 2006; Hayes, Follette, and Linehan 2004; Kabat-Zinn 1990; Kabat-Zinn et al. 1986, 1998; Lutz et al. 2004; Proulx 2003; Rosenbaum, 2007; Roth and Robbins 2004; Williams et al. 2007). It is also actively being applied to the development of attentional skills from preschool to graduate programs (see the appendix).

Relationship to Contemporary Medical Practice

The practice of mindfulness derives from Buddhist tradition, but researchers have adapted it to create behavioral skills that are easily taught and can be broken into smaller components. It has been of great interest to researchers studying its effects on health and performance. The line between scientific inquiry and Buddhist practice blurs at this juncture. Some would make a distinction between mindfulness stripped down to the bare components of attention and mindfulness in Buddhist practice (Wallace 2008).

What is called "mindfulness" in the literature can be defined as the practice whereby a person is intentionally aware of his or her experience in the present moment, nonjudgmentally. It is a conscious moment-to-moment awareness, cultivated by systematically paying attention on purpose in a particular way (Kabat-Zinn 1990, 1994). While mindfulness is a skill involving attention, it is not simply finding a way to distract oneself in order to relax. One could do that by watching television, finding other entertainment, or playing a board game. Rather, this is a practiced skill that increases the capacity to notice where one's attention is without making judgments about either one's attention or the objects themselves. The skill encourages kindness and nonjudgment toward oneself. Rather than a philosophical approach, mindfulness is a demonstrative practice of moment-to-moment awareness that intertwines behaviors with synesthetic perception to settle the mind and emotions, to give rise to resiliency and clarity (Bauer-Wu et al. 2008; Davidson et al. 2003; Williams et al. 2007).

The Center for Mindfulness in Medicine and Society at the University of Massachusetts Medical Center in Worcester, Massachusetts (see appendix), has sponsored courses in so-called mindfulness-based stress reduction (MBSR) and become a clearinghouse for research into the applications that mindfulness can have for adults, teens, and children. Generally speaking, mindfulness practices appear to influence recovery from disability and disease in the areas of pain perception and tolerance, reduce anxiety and depression, diminish the need for analgesics, improve adherence to medical treatments, and show biological effects in neuroendocrine function and immune and autonomic nervous system regulation (Chen et al. 2007; Cooper et al. 2003; Creswell et al. 2007; Davidson et al. 2003; Hanstede, Gidron, and Nyklicek 2008; Hayes, Follette, and Linehan 2004; Lazar et al. 2005; Ludwig and Kabat-Zinn 2008; Lutz et al. 2004; Ott 2002; Resnick, Harris, and Blum 1993; Sitzman, 2002; Speca et al. 2000; see also Linehan in the appendix). Much of this work overlaps with the pioneering work of Herbert Benson (1975) on the relaxation response, which involves composing oneself quietly and paying attention, intentionally, to one's breathing. When distracted by other ideas, concepts, or sounds, one returns one's attention to the breath, purposefully refusing to be distracted by other things that call for attention. Participants may choose a word and repeat it silently over and over, like a mantra. All this is done without judgment toward oneself.

The goal of this method, as in mindfulness meditation (if a goal can be spoken of at all), is greater moment-to-moment awareness. Common side effects (not to be sought directly) of practicing 20 minutes a day are greater relaxation, calmness, and reduction in perceived stress (Benson 1975; Lazar et al. 2000). Studies correlate practice of the relaxation response with increased density of synaptic connections in areas of the brain that mediate attention and emotional regulation (Lazar et al. 2005), as well as changes in autonomic regulation of blood pressure and respiration, while maintaining full oxygen saturation (Dusek et al. 2005). Despite limitations, including small sample size, nongeneralizable effects, and difficulty finding consensus on a working definition of mindfulness, the National Institutes of Health (NIH) now supports studies in an increasing number of varied populations (Ludwig and Kabat-Zinn 2008).

Faith and Culture within Buddhism

Vipassana, or Insight Meditation, by comparison with its Zen siblings, tends to be more meditation-centered, with largely lay participation, gender parity, cross-pollination, and greater social and political engagement (Smith and Novak 2003, p. 43). Japanese Zen, Korean Son, Tibetan Gelug, and Mahayana Pure Land American Buddhist groups tend to have stronger boundaries, hierarchies, and power differences between ordained and lay practitioners. The mixture of these subcultures on U.S. soil can make Buddhist identity difficult to define (Batchelor 1994; Coleman 2000).

In general, Buddhist immigrants to the United States, depending on the country of origin, tend to be concerned less with practicing meditation and more with earning merit, accumulating good karma, and attaining better rebirth through ethical conduct and ritual observance. The laity tend to give respect and prestige to monks (Smith and Novak 2003). Native Buddhist identity derives more from family and culture than from voluntarily taking on the precepts, a step that most Americans take as part of acquiring this new identity. Many immigrants from Cambodia and Vietnam have survived war and genocide; for many of them, the local or regional temple is the center of their

Buddhist culture and life. The performance of religious rituals helps them maintain their connection with their homeland while joining with others here and now in a way that is protective (Balboni et al. 2007; Mollica 2006).

For those sick in the hospital, Buddhist chaplains are foreign to the immigrant Buddhist experience. The normative experience is for family members to ask a monk or nun to pray for the sick person and to chant on that person's behalf—not at the bedside, unless under special circumstances, but in the temple where the *sangha* (community or church) gathers. I work as a family and psychiatric nurse practitioner during the day, and a few evenings a month I work as a Buddhist chaplain at Massachusetts General Hospital in Boston, Massachusetts. As a chaplain I find that native Buddhists often look on me with curiosity and reticence. They may associate even the term *chaplain* with colonialism and Christian missionary work. Their usual question to me is about the temple where I practice. They meet my response with respectful silence when I explain that I practice in the Plum Village tradition of Thich Nhat Hanh with a small sangha that meets in someone's home every Sunday evening.

Buddhist Resources for Living Well

Stories perhaps best illustrate the varied and complex encounters that clinicians and others may have with those who identify as Buddhists. The diversity of encounters is so broad that there is little way to prepare for them except by asking the patient or client about his or her practice—the way that the patient responds to illness, change, and the end of life. I will illustrate engaging with a Buddhist patient's practice with a man whom I saw in the hospital, Mr. McC.

The patient was sure he would not see me again. He had been admitted two days prior, for a disc removal, which was successful. He was healing well, and his wife expected him home on day 3. He had little residual numbness in his right leg, no pain, and his bowels had started to move again. I was visiting Mr. McC because he was on the Buddhist census of the hospital where I made my rounds for the Buddhist chaplaincy. He was born Roman Catholic but had a Buddhist identification. "I am so glad to see you," he said. "I love Thich Nhat Hanh. I have got so much from reading his philosophy. I practice the stuff everyday. He pulled me through this." We parted good company and he was discharged as planned the next day.

Less than four weeks later, I was surprised to find Mr. McC back in the hospital. He had developed a seroma, a fluid-filled sac at the surgical site that led to a systemic infection, and he needed further surgery to clean out the site. He told me, "Everybody and his brother [from the surgical team] have been in to see me to tell me how rare this is. They have been great." It crossed my mind that Mr. McC could have considered a lawsuit, but he was moving in a different direction. To follow the way he was going, I began practicing what is called Insight dialogue, which is a form of Insight meditation. Insight dialogue focuses one in the present moment of a conversation in the same way that Insight meditation focuses one on the present moment of one's breath (Kramer 2007; Susman 2009). Insight dialogue invites the listener to pause, open, relax, trust emergence, listen deeply, and respond honestly. In this case I paused, ignored my considerations of lawsuit, opened and relaxed for a longer conversation.

After listening to him, I shared with him that he could never have predicted or imagined such an outcome when last we met. I offered that not knowing what's going to happen is the heart of impermanence in the Buddhist tradition. He had not thought of impermanence that way, and he agreed that it made sense. Then this insight arose in him: "You never know what is going to happen from one moment to the next. You think you know, but that is just a fabrication of the future." "How often does your fabrication of the future come true?" I asked. He responded, "Maybe 1 percent of the time, if that."

I next shared with him an insight from the Soto Zen teacher Bernie Glassman (1998), who boils the beginning of the whole Zen enterprise down to three interrelated elements. The first is "penetrating the unknown." Mr. McC would never have guessed that he would be back in the hospital. When he accepted this reality, he found himself open to whatever happened next. However, Glassman notes that according to the Buddhist tradition this level of "penetrating the unknown" is not enough. Nonresistance and acceptance of what is must also include a relation-centered attitude. This second element he names "bearing witness," which means looking with others at what is arising in the moment without any judgment or resistance. This may or may not require you to act or do something about the situation with others. The third element is to keep from acting rashly, out of fear or anger; it involves loving action or compassion. You must figure out a response to the changing field using your capacity for loving kindness.

Penetrating the unknown, bearing witness, and loving action were novel to the patient and framed in a helpful way his experience of an unwanted turn of events. In this way, Buddhist practice from a 12th-century Japanese Soto Zen tradition (Dogen, 11th century), communicated by a Buddhist-identified U.S.

chaplain (me), came to shape the experience of a conservative Roman Catholic (Mr. McC) with a mindfulness practice identifying himself as a Buddhist student of Thich Nhat Hanh's lineage (Master Lin Ji, 9th century).

Challenging and Reinforcing Contemporary Medical Practice

Western practitioners may misunderstand the spirituality of native Buddhists and treat them inappropriately as a result.

The mother of my Khmer psychiatric patient was blind and dying in Vietnam. My patient had sent money to have a monk perform a ceremony, but her sister used the money for other purposes. When I empathized with how difficult that must be, my patient disclosed that she was sad and despairing, not about her sister, but about her inability to influence the snakes. "Snakes?" I asked my interpreter. The patient told me that many years ago her mother was tending the garden and killed a snake with her hoe and tossed it away carelessly. As a result, the snake "community" caused her mother to grow blind. The patient needed the ceremony to be performed to correct the insult; this might bring her mother's sight back and save her from going blind. My patient's belief in this instance says less about Buddhist practice and more about folk animistic belief.

Rather than disparage her belief or see this belief as pathological, I asked her to teach me what she believed about the snakes. She explained that in her folk culture, the snake is revered for its role in mediating illness and health between the human community and the more-than-human world. Killing a snake carelessly could subject you to a curse that would cause illness. A monk or shaman could perform specific ceremonies to avoid these consequences (Lavelle et al. 1996). This type of perception is widely known in other cultures as well (Abrams 1996).

As her psychiatric nurse practitioner, I considered the patient's story and her medical record, which noted she had tested glucose intolerant, a prediabetic condition that can be dealt with through diet and exercise. She had been diagnosed with major depression with psychotic features that had resolved with medication. Instead of seeing the patient as having a specific delusion that needed increased medication or attempting to convince her that her mother's blindness probably had to do with diabetes, I set about helping her explore ways that a Buddhist ceremony could be performed here at a local temple. She thought that a temple monk could do it. This allowed us to also consider ways she could take better care of herself through diet and exercise and by volunteering at the temple (altruism), which would bring her closer to her mother, who had once been a temple nun (Wall 2008).

The Harvard Program in Refugee Trauma (HPRT), founded by Richard Mollica, M.D., and James Lavelle, LICSW, has worked with Buddhist refugees from genocide and disaster like this woman for more than 30 years. In his book, Mollica ascribes healing from trauma to human resilience, health promotion, and in particular, acts of altruism and religious ritual performed in community with others. He notes that another significant aspect of healing is the listener's appreciation for a patient's folk beliefs and a willingness to allow the patient to be the teacher or storyteller (Mollica 2006). Both Buddhist communities and programs such as Mollica's have much to teach Western caregivers about healing resources in their culture (see Harvard Program in Refugee Trauma in the appendix).

How Beliefs Influence Practice

Buddhist beliefs inform the practices by which Buddhists deal with not only uncertainty and suffering, but also death. "Can you give this patient the Buddhist last rites?" A well-intended nurse paged the Buddhist chaplain once with this request. There are no "last rites" in Buddhist faith; there is no need because there is only a continuum of life. There is no "last" for there to be a "last" rite. What Buddhists wish for are not the last rites but that the patient be allowed to end life in a quiet, tranquil manner. Honoring this request poses particular challenges for a hospital setting. Yet it invites providers to appreciate the belief that a Buddhist sees clinical death not as the end of life, but as the beginning of a journey that maintains a relationship between the deceased and the family and sangha.

Apart from one's own personal beliefs, honoring this request may convey an empathic connection for the patient and the family that is protective, empowering, and conducive to well-being beyond what the biomedical narrative could provide (Balboni et al. 2007). Yet there are concrete tasks that the dying person and the living community need to complete in assisting the dying to "cross over" and gain a happier rebirth. These tasks make end-of-life care for a Buddhist different from Western practices, which value caring for the dying to the point of death and then leave metaphysical concerns to God or a higher power. Rather than shifting emphasis from the dead body to the bereft community and family, Buddhists try to assist the dying in the transition through death and afterward. Because they value the continued interplay among will, intention, and emotional attachments that have formed personal practice throughout the lifetime, some Buddhists, especially those who meditate, prefer to remain conscious and alert during the process of dying and will not request sedating pain medication. The reason for this is so that they can remain in a state of attention and be able to choose the most preferable realm for rebirth among the many realms that appear in front of one at the time of death, rather than being sedated and vulnerable to emotional turbulence and confusion (Geoffrey DeGraff [Thanissaro Bhikku], Metta Forest Monastery, CA, personal communication, 20 Oct. 2008; DeGraff 2003; Sogyal 2009).

Tibetan Buddhists believe that a lama or a monk may need to assist the dead person to know that his or her bodily form has died and to resolve emotional concerns that may make the passage through death more difficult. However, Tibetans and other Buddhists believe that it is best for the dying not to be touched at time of death. The lama (who can be lay or a monastic teacher) examines the body and carefully touches the crown of the head to awaken the consciousness, refined throughout a lifetime of practice, and allow it to depart through the head. The first place the body is touched determines how the dead person will be reborn. Some believe a lower rebirth results from a touch on the feet than from a touch on the head. Once certain that consciousness has left, the lama declares the person to be dead. This process of departure can last hours, or typically three days after clinical death. During this liminal state, the Tibetan sangha (religious community and family) take up the daily religious practices that the loved one carried out during his or her lifetime, believing that the dying person's habit of practice continues for the person after death. The sangha thus remains in contact with the dead loved one as needed to guide him or her through the journey beyond death to liberation (Lama Migmar Tsetsen, personal communication, 21 Feb. 2009; Lodru 2009; Sogyal 2009).

Nhan Lay was born with a congenital head and spinal cord defect and had survived into adulthood, having escaped the ravages of the Vietnam War with his mother. He could not sit up and needed others to dress and feed him. I met him in his late 20s, when he was hospitalized for surgical decompression of the neck vertebrae. During presurgical admission testing, his doctors found that he had a previously unknown and inoperable ascending aortic aneurysm. What had begun as a simple admission to relieve neck and shoulder pain turned into one focused on end-of-life care. While Nhan Lay was able to come off of a respirator and leave the intensive care unit, the end was only a matter of time.

His mother and sister requested that Nhan Lay not have any chanting done at his bedside out of concern that he would associate it with death and become agitated. Consistent with Buddhist thought, they wanted to avoid agitation and emotional turbulence because these could prevent his consciousness or spirit from moving on at the point of death.

One night when I visited him alone, he lay in bed looking up, unable to speak because of a tracheotomy. I placed my palms together to honor his presence, and he struggled with an IV to touch his small, deformed hands together. He then reached out to take my hand. I found his remarkably warm. He smiled broadly and made a sound like one who is satisfied after a good meal: "mmmm." I said "mmmm" back to him, and we nodded our heads.

Although the family had requested no chanting at his bedside, his mother was a devoted practitioner of the Buddhist Pure Land tradition and had quietly chanted the Great Dharani of Compassion (*Chu Dai-Bi*) many times daily for her son while attending him. On what was to become his death day, the patient agreed to allow my colleague V.L., a Vietnamese Buddhist chaplain, to chant for him during her normal visit. An hour later, the patient died. V.L. came back with J.D., another Buddhist chaplain, for the death service in the patient's room. The patient's mother was sitting by her deceased son, and despite being grief-stricken, she would evoke Namu Amitabha Buddha between her intermittent sobbing. (Amitabha is the cosmic intermediary between Supreme Reality and humankind. Recourse to and faith in Amitabha Buddha promises rebirth in his Paradise.) V.L. set up a small altar with a statue of Sakyamuni Buddha, a small cup of water, some fresh flowers, fruit that was kindly provided by the nursing staff, and incense sticks (unlit due to the general rule of the patient room).

A dozen family members arrived and respectfully requested a Pure Land chanting service. They also brought with them the temple chanting books in Vietnamese. Together amid the sounds of the handbell, V.L. and the family performed the selected traditional chants of the Pure Land for the dead, including the Great Dharani of Compassion (seven times), the Heart Sutra, the Dharani of Pure Land, and most important, the invocation of Namu Amitabha Buddha (*Na Mo A Di Da Phat*), which they did for some five minutes. At the end of the service, several family members sat down by the deceased patient and continuously evoked Namu Amitabha Buddha in a soft tone. Single-mindedly evoking Namu Amitabha Buddha, moment by moment, in the day and in the night, is the essential practice of Pure Land (*Tinh-Do*) tradition (Van Loc Doran, personal communication, 8 Sept. 2009).

The family would continue to do this ritual service every day in the name of the deceased either at home or at temple for 100 days as a collective spiritual prayer for the rebirth of the deceased in the Pure Land of Amitabha Buddha. Pure Land practitioners wish to be reborn in the Pure Land of Amitabha Buddha, also known as the "Land of Pure Happiness" (*Coi Cuc-Lac*), where they will continue their practice toward enlightenment without returning to this suffering world (Nhat Hanh 2003).

Buddhist beliefs and practices have several practical implications for clinicians caring for the dying. Buddhist families benefit from time to anticipate death and for the Tibetan to carry out his ministry that begins after death. At home these religious practices can take place with less tension, but hospitals can try to create a quiet space and offer restful music. Clinicians prescribing pain medication should appreciate the need for the dying person to remain self-aware and to communicate with others, and after death for the bereaved to restrain displays of emotion so as not to interfere with the clinically dead person's inner process.

Addressing and Accessing Spirituality in Practice

The examples described this chapter illustrate the way that I as a Buddhist practitioner incorporate spirituality into my practice as both a Buddhist chaplain and a nurse practitioner. A concluding story of a Buddhist-identified American dealing with death illustrates the latticework of interests that can be present.

Ted and Susan moved in their late 40s from a snug coastal town in Massachusetts, where she had grown up and where they had made their home for 20 years, to the western part of the state because it offered the opportunity for their daughter to attend a better middle school and for them to work with the community of the Insight Meditation Society in Barre, Massachusetts. They were excited to be moving on, finding the sadness of leaving so many years of friendships lessened by their hopes for new beginnings.

A few months after the move, Susan received a diagnosis of pancreatic cancer. Throughout her testing and treatment, she and Ted kept in touch with friends through a Web site where they could exchange news and receive support. A few months after her diagnosis, he posted this poignant and tender reflection on fear, which breathes the spirit of his Vipassana practice:

> The road we have found ourselves on has shown itself to be a prickly one. Life is no longer so simple, little did we know what we could find in our path. Looking back, the past can seem so innocent. Looking forward, the future can appear so ominous. Fear is dressing up in all of its iterations and attempting to convince us that we are at its mercy. It intends to make us brittle. It has a plan to convince us that we are alone, unwanted. As if we were treading water in open ocean, sight of land lost, what happened to the sand we felt between our toes not so long ago? Poor fear, it has no ally in us. It is so uncomfortable in the midst of love. It does not comprehend that we have something else in mind. It is so easily confounded by the presence of courage. We will not banish it, we will invite it to sit a little longer, to rest a bit, breathe with us, look at the unknown, and feel the uncertainty. We ask that it just trust, for a moment, in the possibilities that being awake can provide. We will take it by the hand and share this road. We will show it laughter, compassion, and the love that is growing up all around us. (Ted Sillars, personal communication, 7 Sept. 2009; quoted with permission)

After about a year, Susan was accepted to a hospice and was to move in the day the hospital oncology staff called Ted. They were shocked that he had made this move without consulting the oncologist. Didn't Ted know that there were treatments yet available? Susan needed to be brought immediately to the hospital. Fear in one of its iterations did not comprehend that Ted and Susan had "something else in mind." Yet the oncology team's approach made Ted doubt his decision enough to agree to have her admitted to the hospital to consider all options. Delays and questions raised by specialists diminished those options until she was days from death, too ill to be transferred elsewhere. Family members took turns attending her until she died, without pain, peacefully.

Susan was Jewish with a Vipassana practice. It speaks to the universality of Buddhism that it does not require one to disavow one's own tradition or culture but allows the two traditions to coexist. Ted consulted me about Buddhist funeral rituals. The Plum Village tradition of Thich Nhat Hanh was close to but not exactly like her practice. We kept to her family's traditions of a funeral and burial service officiated by the rabbi, with the associated week-long grieving period of sitting *shiva*. In the spring, a memorial ceremony was held for her at the Insight Meditation Society. The ceremony was neither particularly

Buddhist nor Jewish, but it was Susan's eclectic practice. It provided a joyous way for everyone to remember her together.

I hope the reader will find ways to appreciate Buddhist practice by participating in educational programs in mindfulness, by attending seminars that teach Buddhist practices, or by reading in the subject (Nhat Hanh 1985, 1991). I hope that such appreciation will enhance your interactions when visiting with patients, family, or friends.

It is fitting to conclude this chapter with one of Susan's favorite quotes:

> The good road and the road of difficulties, you have made me cross; and where they cross, the place is holy. (Black Elk of the Oglala Sioux)

APPENDIX

Selected Web Sites for Buddhism, Mindfulness, and Mind/Body

Practice Patterns

The Mindfulness Bell: A Journal of the Art of Mindful Living. www.iamhome.org. A Community for Mindful Living Web site, with Thich Nhat Hanh teachings and a link to a directory of U.S. sanghas.

Zen Peacemakers: A Force for Socially Engaged Buddhism. www.zenpeacemakers.org. "With activities around the globe and a base in Western Massachusetts, the Zen Peacemakers provide training, resources and practice in Socially Engaged Buddhism." Founded by Bernie Glassman.

Upaya Zen Center, Santa Fe, NM. www.upaya.org. Founded by Joan Halifax.

Medicine and Science

Massachusetts General Hospital. Benson-Henry Institute for Mind Body Medicine. www.massgeneral.org/bhi.

Mind and Life Institute. www.mindandlife.org.

University of Massachusetts Medical School. Center for Mindfulness in Medicine, Health Care and Society. www.umassmed.edu/cfm/index.aspx. Includes a link to the Annual Conference on Investigating and Integrating Mindfulness in Medicine, Health Care, and Society.

Mental Health/Trauma

Harvard Program in Refugee Trauma. Richard H. Mollica, director. www.hprt-cambridge.org.

Marsha Linehan, Ph.D. Web site. http://faculty.washington.edu/linehan. Linehan teaches psychology and use of mindfulness training with patients.

Stanford University. Clinically Applied Affective Neuroscience Project. http://caan.stanford

.edu/current_research.html. Research on anxiety and use of mindfulness and cognitive behavioral therapy in adults and children.

Education

ABC National Radio of Australia. Dr. Mindfulness: Science and the Meditation Boom. 10 Nov. 2007. All in the Mind Web site. www.abc.net.au/rn/allinthemind/stories/2007/2082342.htm.

Association for Mindfulness in Education. www.mindfuleducation.org.

Center for Contemplative Mind in Society. www.contemplativemind.org.

Garrison Institute. Contemplation and Education Initiative. www.garrisoninstitute.org.

Inner Kids Mindful Awareness Program. http://susankaisergreenland.com.

Kinder Associates. Wellness Works in Schools. www.mindfulyoga.com/programs/index.htm.

Mindful Awareness Research Center at UCLA. http://marc.ucla.edu.

Mindfulness in Education Network. www.mindfuled.org.

REFERENCES

Abrams, D. 1996. *The Spell of the Sensuous: Perception and Language in a More-than-Human World*. New York: Harcourt.

Baer, R., ed. 2006. *Mindfulness-Based Treatment Approaches: Clinician's Guide to Evidence Base and Applications*. San Diego, CA: Elsevier.

Balboni, T., L. Vanderwerker, S. D. Block, M. Paulk, C. Lathan, J. R. Peteet, and H. Prigerson. 2007. Religiousness and spiritual support among advanced cancer patients and associations with end-of-life treatment preferences and quality of life. *Journal of Clinical Oncology* 24:555–60.

Batchelor, S. 1994. *The Awakening of the West: The Encounter of Buddhism and Western Culture*. Berkeley, CA: Parallax Press.

Bauer-Wu, S., A. M. Sullivan, E. Rosenbaum, M. J. Ott, M. Powell, M. McLoughlin, and M. W. Healey. 2008. Facing the challenges of hematopoietic stem cell transplantation with mindfulness meditation: A pilot study. *Integrative Cancer Therapies* 7:62–69.

Benson, H. 1975. *The Relaxation Response*. New York: Harper Torch.

Chen, E. Y., L. Matthews, C. Allen, J. R. Kuo, and M. M. Linehan. 2007. Dialectical behavior therapy for clients with binge-eating disorder or bulimia nervosa and borderline personality disorder. *International Journal of Eating Disorders* 41:505–12.

Coleman, J. W. 2000. *The New Buddhism: The Western Transformation of an Ancient Tradition*. New York: Oxford University Press.

Cooper, L. M., P. K. Wood, H. K. Orcutt, and A. Albino. 2003. Personality and the predisposition to engage in risky or problem behaviors during adolescence. *Journal of Personality and Social Psychology* 82:390–410.

Creswell, J. D., B. M. Way, N. I. Eisenberger, and M. D. Lieberman. 2007. Neural correlates of dispositional mindfulness during affect labeling. *Psychosomatic Medicine* 69:560–65.

Davidson, R. J., J. Kabat-Zinn, J. Schumacher, M. Rosencrantz, D. Muller, S. F. Santorelli, F. Urbanowski, A. Harrington, K. Bonus, and J. F. Sheridan. 2003. Alterations in brain and immune function produced by mindfulness meditation. *Psychosomatic Medicine* 65:564–70.

DeGraff, G. (aka Thanissaro Bhikku).1993. *The Mind Like Fire Unbound.* Barre, MA: Dhamma Dana Publications.

Dusek, J. A., B. Chang, J. Zaki, J., S. W. Lazar, A. Deykin, G. B. Stefano, A. L. Wohlhueter, P. L. Hibberd, and H. Benson. 2005. Association between oxygen consumption and nitric oxide production during the relaxation response. *Medical Science Monitor* 12:CR1–10.

Glassman, B. 1998. *Bearing Witness: A Zen Master's Lessons in Making Peace.* New York: Bell Tower.

Goldstein, J., and J. Kornfield. 1987. *Seeking the Heart of Wisdom: The Path of Insight Meditation.* Boston: Shambhala Publications.

Hanstede, M., Y. Gidron, and I. Nyklicek. 2008. Effects of a mindfulness intervention on obsessive-compulsive symptoms in a non-clinical student population. *Journal of Nervous and Mental Disease* 196:776–79.

Hayes, S. C., V. M. Follette, and M. M. Linehan, eds. 2004. *Mindfulness and Acceptance: Expanding the Cognitive-Behavioral Tradition.* New York: Guilford Press.

Kabat-Zinn, J. 1990. *Full Catastrophe Living: Using the Wisdom of Your Body and Mind to Face Stress, Pain, and Illness.* 2nd ed. New York: Random House, Bantam Dell.

———. 1994. *Wherever You Go, There You Are: Mindfulness Meditation in Everyday Life.* New York: Hyperion.

Kabat-Zinn, J., L. Lipworth, R. Burney, and W. Sellers. 1986. Four-year follow-up of a meditation-based program for the self-regulation of chronic pain: Treatment outcomes and compliance. *Clinical Journal of Pain.* 2:159–73.

Kabat-Zinn, J., E. Wheeler, T. Light, A. Skillings, M. J. Scharf, T. G. Cropley, D. Hosmer, and J. D. Bernhard. 1998. Influence of a mindfulness meditation-based stress reduction intervention on rates of skin clearing in patients with moderate to severe psoriasis undergoing photo therapy (UVB) and photochemotherapy (PUVA). *Psychosomatic Medicine* 60:625–32.

Kramer, G. 2007. *Insight Dialogue: The Interpersonal Path to Freedom.* Boston: Shambhala Publications.

Lavelle, J., S. Tor, R. F. Mollica, K. Allden, and L. Potts, eds. 1996. *Harvard Guide to Khmer Mental Health.* Cambridge: Harvard Program in Refugee Trauma.

Lazar, S. W., G. Bush, R. L. Gollub, G. L. Fricchione, G. Khalsa, and H. Benson. 2000. Functional brain mapping of the relaxation response and meditation. *NeuroReport* 11:1581–85.

Lazar, S. W., C. E. Kerr, R. H. Wasserman, J. R. Gray, D. N. Greve, M. T. Treadway, M. McGarvey, et al. 2005. Meditation experience is associated with increased cortical thickness. *NeuroReport* 16:1893–97.

Lodru, L. 2009. The Bardos with Lama Lodru Rinpoche. Podcast of a recorded talk. www.upaya.org/dharma/the-bardos (accessed 2 March 2009).

Ludwig, D. S., and J. Kabat-Zinn. 2008. Mindfulness in medicine. *JAMA* 300:1350–52.

Lutz, A., L. L. Greischar, N. B. Rawlings, M. Richard, and R. J. Davidson. 2004. Long-term meditators self-induce high-amplitude gamma synchrony during mental practice. *Proceedings of the National Academy of Science USA* 101:16369–73.

Maezumi, T., and B. Glassman, eds. 2002. *On Zen Practice: Body, Breath, and Mind.* Boston: Wisdom Publications.

Mollica, R. F. 2006. *Healing Invisible Wounds: Paths to Hope and Recovery in a Violent World.* New York: Harcourt.

Nhat Hanh, T. 1985. *A Guide to Walking Meditation.* New Haven: Eastern Press.

———. 1991. *Peace Is Every Step: The Path of Mindfulness in Everyday Life.* New York: Bantam.

———. 1996. *Cultivating the Mind of Love: The Practice of Looking Deeply in the Mahayana Buddhist Tradition.* Berkeley, CA: Parallax Press.

———. 1998. *The Heart of the Buddha's Teaching: Transforming Suffering into Peace, Joy, and Liberation.* New York: Broadway Books.

———. 2003. *Finding Our True Home: Living in the Pure Land Here and Now.* Berkeley, CA: Parallax Press.

Ott, M. J. 2002. Mindfulness meditation in pediatric clinical practice. *Pediatric Nursing* 28:487–91.

Proulx, K. 2003. Integrating mindfulness-based stress reduction. *Holistic Nursing Practice* 17:201–8.

Resnick, M. D., L. J. Harris, and R. W. Blum. 1993. The impact of caring and connectedness on adolescent health and well-being. *Journal of Paediatrics and Child Health* 29:53–59.

Rosenbaum, E. 2007. *Here for Now: Living Well with Cancer through Mindfulness.* Hardwick, MA: Satya House Publications.

Roth, B., and D. Robbins. 2004. Mindfulness-based stress reduction and health-related quality of life: Findings from a bilingual inner-city patient population. *Psychosomatic Medicine* 66:113–23.

Sitzman, K. 2002. Interbeing and mindfulness: A bridge to understanding Jean Watson's theory of human caring. *Nursing Education Perspective* 23:118–23.

Smith, H., and P. Novak. 2003. *Buddhism: A Concise Introduction.* New York: HarperCollins.

Sogyal, R. 2009. *The Tibetan Book of Living and Dying.* San Francisco: HarperCollins.

Speca, M., L. E. Carlson, E. Goddey, and M. Angen. 2000. A randomized, wait-list controlled clinical trial: The effects of a mindfulness meditation-based stress reduction program on mood and symptoms of stress in cancer patients. *Psychosomatic Medicine.* 62:613–22.

Susman, T. 2009. Zen in their bedside manner. *Los Angeles Times*, June 19.

Wall, R. 2008. Healing from war and trauma: Southeast Asians in the US; A Buddhist perspective and the Harvard Program for Refugee Trauma. *Human Architecture: Journal of the Sociology of Self-Knowledge* 6:105–12.

Wallace, A. B. 2008. A mindful balance. *Tricycle Magazine*, Spring. www.alanwallace.org/spr08wallace_comp.pdf (accessed 7 Sept. 2009).

Weiss, A. 2004. *Beginning Mindfulness: Learning the Way of Awareness.* Novato, CA: New World Library.

Williams, M., J. Teasdale, Z. Segal, and J. Kabat-Zinn. 2007. *The Mindful Way through Depression: Freeing Yourself from Chronic Unhappiness.* New York: Guilford Press.

Young, S. 2009. A Pain-Processing Algorithm. www.shinzen.org/Articles/artPainProcessingAlgorithm.pdf (accessed 2 March 2009).

CHAPTER EIGHT

Eclectic Spirituality

Elizabeth Spencer-Smith, M.D., F.A.C.R.

A significant and growing minority of Americans describe themselves as "spiritual but not religious." Their eclectic spirituality (ES) traces the alternate route, the scenic path to the ineffable. The term *eclectic* implies "ideal selection from many sources." Thus, ES involves ongoing study of history's many belief systems, free of the dictates of any. Followers prefer the open-ended to the structured and favor spiritual meandering over settling into one belief. The common thread of ES study is generic spirituality, or spiritual belief per se. But the prime appeal of ES is its focus on mystical and esoteric knowledge, both ancient and modern, especially having to do with arcane, untapped human potential.

ES values the deceptively simple wisdom of ancient shamanism, the world's first religion, currently reemerging as neoshamanism. ES likewise collects more recent spiritual thought from the human potential movements of the latter 20th century, including self-help, New Age, contemplative practice, and humanistic psychology. This melding of ancient and recent wisdom aids navigation of a precarious and complex modern world. Regarding the future of humanity, ES strongly encourages investment in human and global potential by seeking healing belief, overseen by spirit.

Insights about Life and Healing

In ES, any belief that supports well-being amid life's challenges while also promoting both personal growth and the greater good is healing. Pursuit of belief at the expense of other humans is therefore disqualified. ES acknowledges that all the favored "abstracts" of life—personal growth, success, meaning, love, adjustment, sheer understanding, wellness, empowerment, and enlightenment—intertwine with well-being. These variably sought attributes are gained or lost through the choices we make. Sadly, much of human behavior undermines their pursuit, as well as the gains themselves. We fail to realize that we can willfully forge wellness and well-being. In ES, the effort of "tuning the spirit" quickly becomes intriguing, empowering, and fun. But first we must learn to focus attention on well-being per se.

ES espouses the promotion of personal and global well-being through beliefs that engender healthy behaviors, always in concert with nature. Inspired by the healing beauty of the natural world, ES urges a rise above the human condition wherever possible in order to see humanity clearly, especially the sheer impact of human vicious cycles—or why it is that after taking a few steps forward, humans invariably slip more than a few steps back. This remains a compelling human mystery.

ES embraces the entire cosmos throughout time. Any belief, conscious or not, is effected and affected through the interface between our inner and outer worlds. Hence the common ES statements "We are what we believe" and "We create our own reality." Theoretical physics and ES metaphysics often share basic concepts: the biocentric universe theory, recently set forth by Lanza, similarly suggests that human consciousness is the filter that determines what we sense as reality. We "construct" the universe so unconsciously and effectively that it appears as the absolute "out there." What we sense "in here" is exactly the same product (Lanza 2009). String theory postulates subparticular mass-energetic "strings" and 11 dimensions in its current attempt to reconcile the macrocosm (e.g., gravity) with the microcosm, including quantum mechanics. These hypothetical building blocks are reminiscent of the "fibers" of awareness energy and multiple dimensions of shamanism. Einstein spent 30 of his latter years pursuing a unified field theory, an unsuccessful attempt to reconcile general relativity with electromagnetism. Although he explained the behavior of light in detail, he regarded the nature of light as the ultimate mystery (Greene 1999, 2004).

To render the "cosmic" scope of ES manageable, this chapter will be limited to medically relevant "spiritual, not religious" pursuits, including spiritual psychology; spiritual self-help; ancient shamanism and neoshamanism; contemplative practices, including guided imagery; and self-healing principles fostered by the New Thought and New Age movements. Though considered ES "subspecialties," formal mediumship, Reiki, dream work, medical intuitive work, and the like lie afield of evidence-based medicine, where this writing centers. Traditional spiritualities also figure into ES and are covered by other chapters. The attempt here is to embrace and elucidate the broad basics of ES, akin to the general practice of medicine. Indeed, ES shares two basic intents of nearly every medical setting: to heal and to teach self-healing.

A common thread is personal energy efficiency, or impeccability. The practical side of ES urges careful strategy in life, namely, suspending all beliefs and behaviors that waste energy and thereby invite dis-ease, or the stress of human "being," also called existential angst. The greatest human drains seem to stem from the fragile human ego, comprised of a duality: dysfunctional ego (DE) versus functional ego (FE). Functional ego and dysfunctional ego are core beliefs in ES.

After studying what seems a moving nontarget, the ES adherent eventually will narrow his or her field of interest to recurring personal beliefs that ring true. Culling and braiding the abstract into resonant themes demands a holistic thought process, or vision, to be described shortly. For instance, many upstream beliefs have filled my own ES "pool," and they overflow into a semblance of downstream order as 12 core beliefs listed below and described further in subsequent paragraphs. The terms and their context are my own interpretation of a vast body of mostly subjective material.

1. Spirit is an impersonal force called awareness energy (AE), the basic "fiber" of the cosmos, more basic than cosmological particles. "Mass-energy in space-time subject to four basic forces" is one of many interpretations of AE. In the world of spirit, time is compressible (or expandable) through presence and intensity (or lack thereof) (Lanza 2009).
2. Humans are "clusters" of AE connected to each other and with AE at large, or the cosmic fabric. While we seem both separate from the fabric

and divided into mind, heart, body, and soul, humans are simple but unique collections of the same basic fibers of the cosmos; each of us is woven into the cosmic fabric with varying degrees of refinement and alignment (Castaneda 1984; Primack and Abrams 2006).

3. Unconsciousness is rule by instinct and/or by unrefined, unbalanced, or misaligned AE.
4. Consciousness is awareness of awareness (Lanza 2009). Vision, self- and cosmic awareness, presence, clarity, intensity, and sheer understanding are closely related forms of consciousness, or aligned AE (Tolle 2005).
5. The primary human purpose is to grow in awareness, to refine personal AE so as to align with AE at large, a process called enlightenment that eventually culminates in transformation (Castaneda 1984; Walsh and Vaughan 1993).
6. Group AE refinement culminates in a more stable collective transformation and invites the auspicious self-healing prophecy, a shared propitious cycle that eclipses the vicious self-fulfilling prophecy of shared dysfunctional ego (table 8.1, nos. 2, 3, 7, and 8) (Castaneda 1981).
7. The self (ego, life force) is always the sum of aligned, or functional, ego (FE) and misaligned, or dysfunctional, ego (DE). Adding up to one self implies that growth of FE diminishes DE, and vice versa (table 8.1, no. 1).
8. DE dominance means that the individual is ruled by fear of loss of one's illusory sense of control, manifesting as either intense self-reflection or restrictive rationality. DE dominance, literally a self-fulfilling prophecy, is the basic human vicious cycle and may be replaced only by the propitious cycle inherent in the emergence of FE (table 8.1, nos. 2 and 3) (Castaneda 1984).
9. FE dominance equals established vision in place of self-absorption and restrictive rationality. FE manifests as humility, nobility, sobriety, and impeccability, while always relishing life. Because DE is misaligned (distracted or restricted), only FE reaches vision, thereby neutralizing DE in any particular endeavor. FE expands its influence over all personal and collective human endeavors gradually and naturally through self-awareness and positive feedback.
10. FE, on consciously choosing a spiritual link or accepting FE's seamless continuation with the cosmic fabric, becomes higher self (HS),

Table 8.1. Human concept equations in eclectic spirituality

1.	Self (ego, life force) = FE + DE (FE, DE mutually preclusive)
2.	DE dominant self = DE > FE (subconscious vicious cycle → more DE)
3.	FE dominant self = FE > DE (conscious propitious cycle → more FE)
4.	Self-healing AEαFE / DE (self-healing as wellness, well-being, empowerment)[a]
5.	Impeccability = self-healing AE efficiency (hinges on awareness of mortality)
6.	HS = FE linked to higher power or spirit (enabled through vision)
7.	Enlightenment = HS expressed over time → transformation (alignment)
8.	Collective enlightenment = self-healing prophecy (auspicious-propitious cycle)

AE: awareness energy; DE: dysfunctional ego; FE: functional ego; HS: higher self
[a] Self-healing AE is directly proportional to FE and inversely proportional to DE.

one who believes that both acquiescence to spirit and proactive spiritual connection heal and that humans carry the potential for self-healing through this belief. To self-heal, we have to believe (Castaneda 1974). The HS is the master of healing belief (table 8.1, no. 6).

11. Wellness, well-being, and empowerment are the same: self-healing awareness energy, or AE. The degree of self-healing AE available to us is directly proportional to our attainment of FE and inversely proportional to our retention of DE (table 8.1, no. 4).
12. The key to all human success is preserving self-healing AE through impeccability (Castaneda 1987), which is defined as life force efficiency or achievement of awareness of life in the context of death (table 8.1, no. 5; table 8.2, no. 9).

The ES edifice of belief is built on vision. Those adept in ES employ rational, intuitive, and nonrational thought processes equally to establish a body of beliefs about reality. By embracing all three thought processes holistically, they gather and integrate knowledge of the known, unknown, and unknowable realms into a body of experiential wisdom, a process that culminates in overarching, profound vision. An intuitive fusion of self-awareness and cosmic awareness, vision increasingly aligns the believer seamlessly with the cosmic fabric. The special humans who operate from vision naturally and consistently are visionaries, who cultivate their unusual clarity through a sustained sense of presence or being "in the now" (Tolle 2007) and through intensity of focus and purpose. These are all forms of consciousness, which with regular practice becomes enlightenment and culminates in transformation or alignment with spirit. In summary, vision is the key intuition through which all human

Table 8.2. Elements of medical professionalism in eclectic spirituality

1.	Expertise	A healing purpose demands expertise first and foremost.
2.	Detachment	Detachment prevents indulgence in "rescuing" and confrontation. Attachment degrades professionalism and sabotages healing and self-healing.
3.	Empathy	Required in healing compassion, empathy is a transaction, an intentional intuitive "merging" with another's discomfort or difficulty. Sympathy is a reaction, a sham healing that helps only the sympathizer. Patients want empathy and may reject mere sympathy.
4.	Validation	Both a nonverbal and verbal message, validation is communicated empathy. Attitude and tone are the most effective ways to express validation.
5.	Compassion	Compassion is empathy in action and requires gentleness and patience. It is crucial to know the difference between detached compassion and obsessive compassion (obsession = indulgence).
6.	Impeccability	The opposite of indulgence, impeccability is energy efficiency in all aspects of life.
7.	FE expression	DE precludes professionalism; FE entrains it. Suppression of arrogance and reverse arrogance recruits humility, nobility, sobriety, and sense of awe while facing patients and the cosmos.
8.	DE suppression:	DE hides its vulnerability due to fear of inadequacy; likewise, DE basks in self-importance. Medical professionalism requires suppression of false bravado and all other DE "blinders."
9.	Death perception	True professionals have gained intimate awareness of life in the context of death. To operate as if one is immortal is to squander resources, degrade impeccability, and undermine excellence.

DE: dysfunctional ego; FE: functional ego

thought ultimately connects to the sheer mystery of the unknowable, or spirit. Indeed, the unknowable cannot be described, but only experienced through growing personal and collective vision.

ES seeks balance between the subjective and the objective. It urges us to choose paths that entice us (toward the unknown), while remaining realistic (aware of the known) and deeply mindful of spiritual presence (the unknowable). To select a path, we must learn to trust our feelings. But as a rule, we humans first perceive, then believe, and thence conceive emotions; thus the importance of the perception-belief process, also termed "attention." In making choices, we must also realize that our emotions can directly influence our perceptions and thoughts about them. Moreover, ES informs us that not all feelings arise from human attention and that spirit is constantly sending direct emotional messages—called omens, signs, and healing grace—Jungian synchronicities (Jung 1959) that become more evident and frequent as vision unfolds. Because we are taught young to focus our attention mostly on the known, most of us miss or misinterpret these subtle cues. In the last analysis, ES invites all healing beliefs and the emotions they evoke to explain our essential nature, yet always urges rationality for this purpose, thereby encouraging fully integrated healing, manifested in holistically healing attitudes and behaviors.

Turning now to the practical, ES compels us to rise above the human ego's restricted awareness to see its flaws from a higher context—specifically, to acquire vision in place of self-absorption and restrictive rationality. Vision discloses these flaws as reversible "snags" in human awareness energy (AE), as simple misalignments related to our belief-set anchored in unconsciousness. Thus, the thrust of the practical message of ES is that the distortion called dysfunctional ego (DE) is the seminal human flaw—primarily because DE precludes the development of functional ego (FE), the "true self," the only facet of human AE capable of forging a tenable path to healing, self-healing, and spiritual connection.

In ES, we begin to master our dysfunctional beliefs and behaviors when we achieve awareness of them. Vision further reveals that DE indulgence has two different AE "twists." Self-absorbed DE is obsessed with an entirely self-invented notion called self-image and spends most of its thrust—essentially our time and energy—rallying around this phantom projection. Restrictive DE likewise curtails human awareness through a special form of denial called "seeing is believing," or insistence on reason alone to explain reality. Both are unhealthy configurations of human AE because they promote obsession with the known to the exclusion of the far more empowering unknown and unknowable realms (Castaneda 1984). Thus, we miss out on the intrigue of the unknown and we fail to acquire the sobriety, humility, perspective, and wisdom linked to the unknowable. DE forces this separation without our knowledge, the way its compelling undercurrents have dominated human AE for eons. The only exception to DE's restrictive rationality occurs on choosing spiritual belief. But such a connection proves tentative because of DE "attachments" to fear, self-image, or personal gain.

Just as we learned young, from our parents, role models, and peers to "create" a restricted reality, we likewise imprinted DE as "normal" human nature. We all were taught the DE dominant worldview before we can remember, and in turn we teach it to our young. We subliminally deny the impact of DE dominance, tending to assume that our current human nature is stamped in our genes. DE also escapes our detection through yet another subversive tactic: projection of personal dysfunctions on others rather than owning up to them ourselves.

While on the cosmic scale DE is a minor twist in the flow of AE, on human terms DE is a vicious, self-feeding entrapment that paralyzes human potential. DE dominance, equivalent to original sin in Christianity and other spiritualities, can also be thought of as just a trap we fell into, perhaps out of intense fear of the immensity of the unknown, a self-protective recoiling from our first rational glimpse of the eternity around us (Castaneda 1984).

Relationship to Contemporary Medical Practice

ES challenges medicine by asserting that it places too much emphasis on "patch-up" and not enough on addressing health-eroding beliefs and behaviors. Our treatment guidelines mostly fail to address human nature as the ultimate cause of dis-ease. ES urges a "divine rewrite" here: medicine must strongly consider changing its restrictive, mostly subliminal belief-set regarding human potential. It is time to entertain the possibility that humans can learn to self-heal and that self-healing is truly worth the effort. Surgeons-general Luther L. Terry and C. Everett Koop both attached their reputations to a healing vision of a smoke-free society—a bold belief that started with Terry's confidence in humanity's ability to change.

ES supports the evidence-based method as providing the most reliable set of tools with which to accomplish the miracles of medical science. At the same time, ES challenges the bias of evidence-based medicine against the use of the placebo effect—the hidden power of expectation shared by patient and physician. Most physicians in practice eventually come to appreciate the power of the placebo and see that it has remained fully operative in medicine all along, either subconsciously or behind the examining room door. ES recognizes that conscious belief is only the tip of the iceberg; subconscious belief is pervasive and powerful, and rules.

Subconscious belief may be unconscious (instinctual) or subliminal (denied). If it supports healing and erases doubt (such as by fostering trust in a healer or treatment), subconscious belief may aid the healing process. If misdirected or conflicted, subconscious belief may negate healing directly or generate angst that distracts or depletes healing. ES claims that bringing subconscious belief into full awareness can only help—by releasing and allowing this energy to align with healing purpose and higher order (one and the same in ES). So perhaps the next logical step for evidence-based physicians is to develop ways to harness the placebo effect consciously, ethically, in full disclosure—by exposing and defusing its nonhealing potential based in fear, while promoting its healing potential anchored in faith and trust. But first we must rebuild conscious belief in the power of belief.

The emphases of conventional medicine and ES converge in the recovery programs of addiction medicine, which share features of spiritual psychology. Other chronic diseases, especially those that profoundly challenge a patient's ability to cope—fibromyalgia, obesity, depression, and chronic pain—also may benefit from recovery programs that promote scientific holism (Martinez-Lavin 2008) and visionary connection to a higher concept.

Struggles of Believers with Contemporary Medical Practice

Acute illness in rheumatology, my field, can be frightening because such diseases are often systemic and produce many odd and painful symptoms. The case I remember most vividly is that of a spiritually minded, supremely health-conscious male in his early 50s who presented with the sudden onset of joint pain and swelling, along with a positive rheumatoid arthritis test, meeting the diagnostic criteria for acute rheumatoid arthritis (RA). He first expressed disbelief on hearing the diagnosis because, he said, "I have been so careful about my health." A detailed history excluded other autoimmune features in the patient and his family and failed to identify any stressors or maladaptive behaviors. The unusual aspect of his presentation was that he already had researched and diagnosed his disease; in fact, he had read of recent "cures" using antibiotics in early RA and wanted to try one of the tetracyclines (which were marginally evidence-based treatments then, and are now overshadowed by far more effective regimens). I went along with his request as a reasonable temporizing measure while waiting for additional tests. I asked him to return in two weeks because his disease was rather aggressive.

He returned six months later, and only for my benefit, to report that he was entirely free of joint pain and swelling. The arthritis had disappeared completely after he had taken the antibiotic for just a few weeks. He was sure that intensifying his spiritual practice had helped. I refrained from bringing up the possibility that he had either viral arthritis or "palindromic" RA (intermittent RA flares that can return at any time). Instead, I wholeheartedly congratulated him for healing himself, because, in an ES sense, he had.

At first, ES adherents with acute illness may be baffled, even shocked, and tend to misinterpret illness as failure of consciousness, thus adding further burden to their setback—but not for long. Growing consciousness forges subconscious resilience, the subliminal capacity to cope that surprises everyone. This ES-minded patient had trained himself to deal with fear and other negative emotions as indicators of maladaptive belief. He remembered that adversity is a challenge rather than a curse and carries a message. Instead of succumbing to fear, guilt, and shame, he chose responsibility and belief in the chance of a cure, even though remote. He initiated self-healing through his own evidence-based research while redoubling efforts to align his awareness with healing belief or faith in a positive outcome. He requested an innocuous traditional medication and believed in it. Even though the antibiotic most likely served as a placebo, I chose not to "contaminate" his self-healing triumph with my rational beliefs because they could elicit a negative expectation for the future.

Many ES patients who have chronic illness are secondarily inspired after they receive the diagnosis. Others, though ensconced in ES, develop a chronic disease despite having moved toward healthier beliefs and behaviors. I have observed both phenomena, mostly the former. Patients who have a chronic disease in general seem genuinely interested in how they can help themselves, often focusing first on diet and supplements. The strategy to favor with ES-minded and growth-oriented patients is to reinforce their belief that negative emotions such as depression, disappointment, guilt, and shame only compound problems. I often will declare, "What's done is done and we can't go back, so why not move forward?" It takes time for the patient to adjust to the new paradigm called chronic disease, but the process goes much faster with vision.

The subject of complementary and alternative treatment (CAM) strikes a personal chord because I have practiced rheumatology in various localities nationwide and have observed nearly all patients employing these modalities to varying degrees. The folk remedies tried for arthritis are legion and are unlikely to go away. The tenacious preference for CAM in human disease seems to stem from the sufferer's denial of illness, fear of pharmacologic side effects, desire for a sense of control, problems with access to care, and highly effective marketing. But my bias is that patients in general, and ES-minded patients in particular, value self-reliance and simply want to try self-healing first. ES understands that science and belief complement each other. But the credibility of CAM remains questionable due to an overemphasis on unproven products. CAM offers them as "natural" (what is that?) and "alternative" (i.e., given for alternative's sake). Both claims are not only illogical but also subversive due to subtle bias against proven treatments. Many patients choose this road and delay proper care, often burning bridges back to wellness. A few formerly scientific physicians have chosen it too—for both nonrational and (horrors!) entrepreneurial reasons. CAM is overdue for a rational overhaul.

In contrast, ES espouses proven treatments plus "alternative" beliefs and behaviors to complement science and prevent the need for medical treatment in the first place. ES suggests that this may be achieved by teaching patients how to pursue personal impeccability. In addition, ES considers all potential healing belief, especially generic spirituality, ripe for scientific study through analysis of behavioral change and health outcomes associated with belief.

Occasionally a patient who has cancer will appear in a rheumatology practice as a diagnostic dilemma. The following patient proved much more than that. He was a man in his 30s, slender and muscular, sporting an orange glow. He was committed to meditation and enlightenment through consciousness, and this somehow had translated into ardent health-consciousness. Referred by his primary physician for evaluation of severe back pain, he gave unmistakable clues that the pain was not musculoskeletal. A detailed history disclosed a 10-pound weight loss, although he had attributed it to stepping up his exercise program, thinking that doing so might help his back. In addition, he was taking one of the most varied and extensive arrays of supplements and esoteric health concoctions I had ever come across. The orange dermis was due to a massive excess of carotenoids, not jaundice. The patient was also taking several different "blends" of alfalfa sprouts containing emulsified sprouts plus many mostly unidentifiable ingredients, unaware of a current rumor that alfalfa sprouts might cause cancer.

Unfortunately, tests showed that his liver enzymes were highly abnormal. By CT scan and biopsy, the patient turned out to have a large liver cancer, inoperable and virtually untreatable, having metastasized. So this was a sporadic case of untreatable cancer in an unfortunate man in his prime. His angst and sadness on learning of his plight overwhelmed all of his caregivers, primarily because none of us could give him an answer as to "Why me, when I have been so health-conscious?" No one made any attempt to address his obsession with supplements and the implicit psychological issues, nor did we give any hint that something he took could have stimulated the tumor. There was no point and no proof. He died shortly thereafter, leaving a young family.

I recall my eerie suspicion at the time that those who cling so tightly to life may be prescient. But I also toyed with the possibility that the clinging (the fear) is what bled his life force (i.e., through inexorable self-fulfilling prophecy). Fear and the need to control it (fear of fear) are lethal taskmasters. Creative speculation concerning the unknowable is never rational, yet I retain the belief that excessive supplementation with randomly selected, unproven, potentially harmful substances is illogical and indicative of blind fear, the archenemy of healing.

People caught up in blind fear must learn to love this miracle called life, to trust that there is natural healing built into to our life force, and to master "taking control by letting go," an ES behavioral trademark.

How Beliefs Influence Practice

The misconception that human nature is incorrigible is tenacious. It is difficult to convince anyone, even the enlightened at times, to the contrary because we all read the headlines. Yet the ES-minded, who recognize that humans suffer from their shared unconsciousness, are not impatient, frustrated, or jaded because we once shared fully in the DE mindset and understand that consciousness emerges on its own schedule.

ES seeks solutions, not just "kneading the bad news." Simple education would go a long way toward solving the majority of problems in health care. But for individuals who are narcissistic or who are in relationships dominated by DE (DE-DE relationships), more intensive "higher education" is required. These are major challenges for most humans and stem from the same problem, DE dominance. Narcissism, according to ES vision, is 100 percent DE—implying that narcissists focus only on the realm of the known. Castaneda's Don Juan called them "petty tyrants," people driven to obsessively manipulate a narrow worldview called self-absorption. They are unaware of any other view, especially that of other people (Castaneda 1984). Nor can they fathom the unknown and unknowable realms with any sense of awe. The narcissist is stuck at age two. In various facets, we all are narcissists due to our subtle programming. Only the impeccable warrior against the self can become fully free (Campbell 1973). By definition, all DE-DE relationships deteriorate into significant "bilateral" narcissism. So ES concludes that narcissism in varying degrees is the seminal unsolved human problem—one that freely invites dis-ease, and therefore much of human disease and premature aging.

ES patients, often highly successful professionals, are pleasant and reasonable because they are always working on their personal "issues." ES patients are proactive regarding health maintenance and researching disease treatments. Rather than feel preempted, their physicians may do well to read some of their patients' information. A patient of mine who has severe fibromyalgia hands me the results of his Internet searches at most visits; I try to find time to study them. Recently a new drug for fibromyalgia was released; he had informed me about it five years ago! Interestingly, this patient lost his young son many years ago; the subject is still too painful for him to discuss. He has declined treatment for post-traumatic stress disorder despite referrals. Instead, he focuses on the pain and the possibility for a scientific cure. Even though he is medically sophisticated and "spiritual, not religious" (Heckel 2008), he seems blocked in a crucial area. I have acknowledged this and still do what I can to help him. We all become stuck in various facets and may never find our way out of certain snags. But the ES idea is to try anyway, because as a rule becoming more conscious can only help. In this patient's case, the cycle of psychic pain, fear, and denial seems too deeply engrained for him to escape it. But there always is hope.

Narcissistic patients always manage to challenge physicians and their staffs to the core. We shudder on seeing certain names on the schedule. But narcissistic physicians may do far greater damage. Overt intimidation (bullying) and subtle manipulation (gossip, backstabbing, one-upmanship) are problems in medical schools and among physicians in practice. Although most physicians would like to think otherwise, we are imprinted with the current version of human nature like everyone else. However, we tend to hide ours behind the white coat of altruism. Even though considered members of a noble profession, we physicians are only as strong as our weakest, most narcissistic links—both as a group and as individuals. The only way to deal with narcissism is to meet it head on and quell it with professionalism and honesty. Though it seems impossible when facing a bullying or subtly manipulative narcissist, ES suggests we muster the requisite professionalism by empathizing with the narcissist's plight. In the final analysis, narcissism in others serves as a convenient mirror for our own: Whatever repels us in others often is a muted cry for self-awareness of the same issue lurking within.

ES identifies yet another potential DE trap common to medicine: Some caregivers are so busy helping others that they forget to care for themselves. This is called "obsessive compassion," as opposed to the more professional "detached compassion" (table 8.2, no. 5). These caregivers succumb to a hidden delusion called indispensability, the DE trait that stems from self-importance. Contrary to DE fantasy, the world drives right on by when the indispensable run out of gas.

Medical professionalism is a collection of ideals (see table 8.2). Few physicians possess the time and motivation to work on their own DE. We enjoy our well-earned status and often take a pass on growth beyond our requisite schooling, extensive training, and continuing medical education well into our elder years. There are, of course, exceptions: the rare physician choosing enlightenment as a life purpose, with medical practice providing the spiritual path. Even more rare are the special souls who started out in life inspired to "do the right thing in everything" and who continue to orbit this basic stance their entire practice lives, invariably attracting a lifelong following.

Faith and Culture

Much of ES resonates with ancient and neoshamanism. Shamanism was the first spiritual belief system, arising spontaneously on six of seven continents at least 20,000 years ago with surprisingly uniform beliefs and practices. Migration alone does not explain its widespread presence, one of our oldest mysteries. Moreover, because shamans are healers as well as spiritual mediators, shamanism is the world's oldest healing profession. Ancient shamanism retreated "underground" centuries ago to survive the darker aspects of the emerging great religions (Walsh 2007). It reappeared in modern times with the rise of anthropology, specifically the scholarly work of Mircea Eliade (1964).

Studying shamanic culture is difficult without a degree of participation, which then compromises objectivity. The extended works of Castaneda, based on anthropologic fieldwork he began in 1960, exemplify "soft" scholarship and remain highly controversial. (He participated fully as an apprentice shaman, writing 12 best-selling books about the experience.) Yet his work enticed many to the Native American shamanic fold, unearthing forgotten human truths and hidden human potential through the intriguing teachings of Don Juan, a Yaqui Indian shaman living in Arizona and Mexico (Castaneda 1972–87). Despite its questionable academic credibility, many choose to follow the wisdom codified in the Castaneda series.

Neoshamanism thus arose in the wake of the great societal rupture of the latter 20th century. The messy and unruly "revolution" of the 1960s found a large portion of the younger generation abandoning organized religion (Wuthnow 1998). Many looked to shamanism as an alternative discipline (Walsh 2007). However, "liberated" Western culture misappropriated shamanic ritual as license to indulge in drug use for entertainment; our society is still paying dearly for this mistake. As Castaneda later discovered, traditional shamanic mind-altering drugs are strictly supervised and used only briefly as growth tools for a select few on the path to knowledge. Most who are adept do pursue altered states in order to heal and self-heal, but mainly through natural, safer means, such as behavioral control, meditation, movement practice, drumming, dreaming, channeling, and gazing (Walsh 2007). While ancient shamanism encompassed entire cognitive systems of intertwining faith and culture, ES in general and neoshamanism in particular are untraditional and esoteric, and thus separate from present-day culture.

Addressing and Accessing Spirituality in Practice

Appropriate attitude and tone create a "sacred space" in which to share healing expertise. In fact, a careful blend of attitude, tone, and expertise is the key to influencing all matters human. It is up to the physician to nurture a caring attitude and healing tone. Studying ES has enhanced my attitude and approach to medicine, and to life, in the following ways:

1. To diagnosis an illness, I often will intuit or "merge with" the patient's symptoms and test results. This requires a blank mind (i.e., removing all bias and "noise"). The answer—a differential diagnosis or reasonable treatment—will soon appear in my mind's eye. If it does not, I assiduously reexamine and rethink. This "trick" of seeking an intuitive "alignment" of the patient's and the physician's awareness energy (AE) seems to open a "channel" for healing. I do not mean to imply that science is secondary, just that this is a method for applying extensive knowledge to an individual patient's presentation.

2. To manage chronic disease, I first urge the patient to acknowledge (never accept) the illness—a self-healing act in itself (Leech and Singer 1988). To facilitate this task, I suggest that the patient view illness as a loss calling for a classic five-stage grief process (Kubler-Ross 1969). Then I recommend imagining a similar "channel" for healing through the same "wound" (Rossman 2000).
3. My next priority is to address patients' blind fear with scientific information and recognition of fear as a problem in itself. It is important to co-strategize an approach that recognizes reasonable fears and dispels unreasonable ones. I consider fear management crucial to disease management; ideally, it begins on the very first visit.
4. I approach patient care with less trepidation and defensiveness because I have come to see myself as a healer and a physician. I have learned that both titles demand humility and that physicians cannot truly heal until they have learned to heal themselves. A physician-patient relationship can promote growth and healing for both parties (Walsh 2007).
5. In place of micromanaging patients, I have learned to "take control by letting go," supporting medical recommendations with science wherever possible.
6. I take advantage of the fact that faith in a positive outcome is contagious. There is little reason for physicians to back-pedal proven treatments. Moreover, describing positive results in previous patients paves the way for the current patient to forge rational healing belief based on the physician's experience.
7. I consider stress a precursor to disease and premature aging (Miller 2009). Stress depletes and destabilizes our energies, resulting in a loss of center and a disconnection from natural healing AE. Illness or addiction may arise from this energy depletion. Patients are often aware of the ravages of stress but may have little awareness of their personal energies until taught to intuit and nurture them.
8. To tap spirituality as a healing strategy, if the time and place call for it, I will ask the patient off-handedly, "What are your spiritual leanings? The reason why I ask is that in many studies spiritual belief has been associated with better outcomes." I may add the qualification, "I am not espousing a particular belief, just considering all avenues." If the patient is spiritual, I encourage reinforcing the spiritual connection, faith in a positive outcome, belief in evidence-based medicine, and belief in the

healing power of all three. I introduce these after approaching the medical problem scientifically. I subtly remind the patient that positive emotions such as hope, optimism, confidence, and faith only help.

9. If the patient is not spiritual, I concentrate on secular ways to allay fear and promote trust. These include the aspects of professionalism listed in table 8.2, and encouragements to be optimistic, such as "Let's invest in a positive outcome" or "It is important to have faith."
10. I never recommend forging a new spiritual connection as part of a treatment strategy, although I discuss the fact that many studies demonstrate the health benefits of spiritual belief. Most patients accept this as intuitively true. Regarding prayer, I am uncomfortable praying with patients in the traditional manner. Prayer in ES is a proactive engagement with spirit called affirmation. It is neither an invocation nor a supplication because both seem inconsistent with spirit being an impersonal force. Affirmation is a property of will. I "affirm" with every patient I see by rising into professionalism through FE as best I can, by "channeling" and sharing healing information, and then by literally "willing" patients to heal, often out loud.
11. As part of my own quest to better handle narcissism (including my own), I teach patients how to prevent stress by identifying narcissism sooner and dealing with it impeccably (table 8.1, no. 5). Other resources for self-healing include personal resource management (Spencer-Smith 2006); promotion of abundant, balanced, centered, connected energy (ABCC, discussed next); assumption of responsibility for wellness and behavioral accountability; seeking illness meaning; regarding life as opportunity for growth; and respecting death as the ultimate challenger of life. I frequently find myself saying to patients, "As I offer you this advice, I am talking to myself."
12. I instruct patients on how to maximize ABCC energy in the following ways: (a) attention to physical well-being (exercise, diet, and rest); (b) impeccable approach to all of life; (c) pursuit of passions, predilections, talents, and life purpose; (d) avoidance of imbalance and all indulgence; (e) centeredness within any higher concept; (f) pursuit of synergistic (FE-FE) connections; and (g) transformation of adversity into opportunity with the attitude that "there are no mistakes, just learning experiences."
13. I remind myself that DE is tenacious, even in those who are conscious.

DE slips will always occur, as will tests of self-awareness and of our capacity to forgive both self and others (Karen 2001).

Conclusion

ES is an esoteric "nonsystem" of belief both spiritual and practical with meandering emphasis. Progress in ES hinges on the adept's ability to take control by letting go and to acquiesce to the promptings of the ineffable. Success in ES is defined by wellness, well-being, and empowerment under all life circumstances, enabled and sustained through relentless pursuit of personal impeccability. "The trick is in what one emphasizes," says Castaneda's Don Juan. "We either make ourselves miserable, or we make ourselves strong. The amount of work is the same" (Castaneda 1972, p. 184).

REFERENCES

Campbell, J. 1973. *The Hero with a Thousand Faces*. Princeton: Princeton University Press.

Castaneda, C. 1972. *Journey to Ixtlan: The Lessons of Don Juan*. New York: Washington Square Press.

———. 1974. *Tales of Power*. New York: Washington Square Press.

———. 1981. *The Eagle's Gift*. New York: Simon and Schuster.

———. 1984. *The Fire from Within*. New York: Simon and Schuster.

———. 1987. *The Power of Silence: Further Lessons of Don Juan*. New York: Washington Square Press.

Eliade, M. 1964. *Shamanism: Archaic Techniques of Ecstasy*. Princeton: Princeton University Press.

Greene, B. 1999. *The Elegant Universe: Superstrings, Hidden Dimensions, and the Quest for the Ultimate Theory*. New York: Norton.

———. 2004. *The Fabric of the Cosmos: Space, Time and the Texture of Reality*. New York: Knopf.

Heckel, A. 2008. More describe selves as spiritual, not religious. *Daily Camera* (Boulder, CO), 27 April.

Jung, C. G. 1959. *Basic Writings of C. G. Jung*. New York: Modern Library.

Karen, R. 2001. *The Forgiving Self: The Road from Resentment to Connection*. New York: Anchor Books.

Kubler-Ross, E. 1969. *On Death and Dying*. New York: Simon and Schuster/Touchstone.

Lanza, R. 2009. *Biocentrism: How Life and Consciousness Are the Keys to Understanding the True Nature of the Universe*. With B. Berman. Dallas, TX: Benbella Books.

Leech, P., and Singer, Z. 1988. *Acknowledgement: Opening to the Grief of Unacceptable Loss*. Laytonville, CA: Wintercreek Publications.

Martinez-Lavin, M. 2008. Fibromyalgia conundrum: Is scientific holism the answer? *The Rheumatologist* 2:26–27.

Miller, M. 2009. Type D personality traits can hurt heart health. *Harvard Mental Health Letter*, Nov.

Primack, J., and N. E. Abrams. 2006. *The View from the Center of the Universe: Discovering Our Extraordinary Place in the Cosmos.* New York: Riverhead Books.

Rossman, M. 2000. *Guided Imagery for Self-Healing: An Essential Resource for Anyone Seeking Wellness.* Novato, CA: New World Library.

Spencer-Smith, E. 2006. Personal resource management: A "Spirituality and Healing in Medicine" course handout (unpublished) available through the course director at Harvard Medical School: naxelrod@partners.org.

Tolle, E. 2005. *A New Earth: Awakening to Your Life's Purpose.* New York: Plume.

Walsh, R. 2007. *The World of Shamans: New Views of an Ancient Tradition.* Woodbury, MN: Llewellyn.

Walsh, R., and F. Vaughan, eds. 1993. *Paths beyond Ego. The Transpersonal Vision.* New York: Tarcher/Putnam.

Wuthnow, R. 1998. *After Heaven: Spirituality in America since the 1950s.* Berkeley and Los Angeles: University of California Press.

CHAPTER NINE

Christian Science

Christine J. Driessen, C.S.B., M.A., M.S.T., J.D.

Genesis 1, the beginning of the Christian and Jewish Scripture, states that Spirit alone has created all and made everything good and that Spirit made each of us, man or woman, in the divine image and likeness. Mary Baker Eddy, the founder of Christian Science, found this to be a scientific basis for prayer, enabling anyone to prove that health is our natural state.

Christian Science is the universal system of Mind-healing (Mind meaning God, the divine creative intelligence of the universe) through the understanding of the omnipotence and supremacy of Spirit as the source of all creation. It is based on the teachings and healing work of arguably the greatest physician who ever lived, the Jewish teacher Jesus, called the Christ or the Messiah.

Through spiritual means alone, Jesus healed every type of physical condition (Matthew 4:23–24)—acute and chronic; contagious, congenital, hereditary; even long-standing conditions: a woman whose bleeding continued unabated for 12 years in spite of medical treatment (Mark 5:25–34); a woman bowed over, unable to stand erect for 18 years (Luke 13:11–17); a long-standing case of epilepsy (Matthew 17:14–21; Mark 9:14–29); and a man unable to walk for 38 years (John 5:2–9). Jesus resuscitated people who had already died—a

12-year-old girl (Mark 5:21–24, 35–43); a young man being carried to his tomb (Luke 7:12–16); his friend Lazarus, who had been dead for four days (John 11:1–44)—all healed instantly through prayer based on his acknowledgment that God, Spirit, is our only Life (John 11; Matthew 12:22–28).

Jesus taught that anyone who followed his teaching would be able to heal as he did and do even greater works (John 14:12). His command to his followers was, "Heal the sick, cleanse the lepers, raise the dead, cast out devils; freely ye have received, freely give" (Matthew 10:8). "These signs will follow those who believe; in my name they will cast out demons; . . . they will lay hands on the sick, and they will recover" (Mark 16:17, 18; biblical quotations from Kohlenberger 2004).[1] Through his healing work, Jesus defined the meaning of "Christ" as a universal saving power (Luke 7:19–22). Hebrew prophets such as Moses, Elijah, and Elisha, and the disciples of Jesus (in particular, Peter, Paul, and John) all demonstrated the power of Spirit to heal disease and overcome death.

Eddy called this system of healing "Science" because a science is truth or knowledge based on universal laws that anyone can test or put into practice when the laws are understood (such as the science of mathematics). Christian Science refers to the divine laws of Life, Truth, and Love found in the Bible which govern the universe, including each of us irrespective of religious background, and which can be tested and proven by anyone who adheres to them (Eddy 1906, p. 107).

These laws declare that our reason for existing is to glorify God, not through suffering, but by demonstrating our inherent wholeness as God's creation. Eddy explains our purpose: "As an active portion of one stupendous whole, goodness identifies man with universal good. Thus may each member of this church rise above the oft-repeated inquiry, What am I? to the scientific response: I am able to impart truth, health, and happiness, and this is my rock of salvation and my reason for existing" (1913, p. 165).

Eddy called this the "Science of the Christ" or "Christian Science" because "Christ" and "Christian" refer to the healing power of divine Love as demonstrated by Jesus. His life and teaching illustrate how obedience to the two great commandments found in Judaism, Christianity, and Islam—"Love (trust, obey, submit to) God, Spirit, supremely," and "Love your neighbor as yourself"—will enable anyone to heal as he did and prove that our life is entirely spiritual here and now.

The Bible has many references to the "Science of God,"[2] which it describes as perfect and accessible through the Christ. The Bible warns against false science, which it defines as any teaching that steers people away from faith in God, Spirit, as the only power. Eddy also called Christian Science "Mind healing," referring not to the brain—which can be injured, unconscious, or in a coma—but to the one ever-present, all-knowing, divine Mind, God, which enabled Jesus to heal. The apostle Paul said we need to have the Mind of Christ.

Insights about Life and Healing

Christian Science is both therapeutic and preventive, and it declares that health, peace, and wholeness are natural to each of us eternally: "The Christian Science God is universal, eternal, divine Love, which changeth not and causeth no evil, disease, nor death" (Eddy 1906, p. 140). Rather than holding an anthropomorphic concept of God, Eddy believed the God of the Bible to be all-powerful, all-knowing, all-acting; the only creator and the source of good alone, whose law supports and maintains all creation; the All-in-all or sine qua non of existence.

Her insights came from years of searching for better health for herself. After suffering from digestive and back problems, she tried allopathic medicine, homeopathy, and many forms of alternative medicine available during her lifetime but could find no permanent relief. Her discovery of a reliable system of healing came in stages, after a period of experimenting with homeopathic medicine and prayer to treat disease (Eddy 1906, p. 152).

When she cured a woman who had dropsy (edema), whom doctors had abandoned, simply by administering what today would be called a placebo (Eddy 1906, p. 156), she began to appreciate the mental nature of all suffering. However, it was not until she experienced a serious fall and her own healing through prayer alone that she understood its full significance. She wrote: "During twenty years prior to my discovery I had been trying to trace all physical effects to a mental cause; and in the latter part of 1866 I gained the scientific certainty that all causation was Mind [God, Spirit], and every effect a mental phenomenon. My immediate recovery from the effects of an injury caused by an accident, an injury that neither medicine nor surgery could reach, was the falling apple that led me to the discovery how to be well myself, and how to make others so" (1892, p. 24).

Eddy discovered in Genesis 1 an explanation for how Jesus healed and how she was healed. This chapter explains that Spirit created the entire universe, but there is no mention of evil, disease, sin, or death in creation. Genesis 1:26–

27 states that man ("male and female") is given dominion over all the earth. (Jesus demonstrated that this "dominion" is our ability to prove the omnipotence of Spirit here in the human experience through healing.) Deuteronomy 32:4 declares God's work to be perfect. Ecclesiastes 3:14 says that God's work is forever; nothing can be added to it or taken from it, so it is logical to assume that disease cannot be added to God's creation, nor can dishonesty, hate, stress, malfunctioning, or failure. And normal action, proper growth, and right thinking cannot be taken away from it.

The explanation for why suffering, disease, aging, accident, and death seem real and inevitable is found in another scriptural narrative, Genesis 2 and 3, the allegory of Adam and Eve. This second version of creation is entirely material; the creator is neither all-knowing nor all-powerful; and the creation is something of a failure from the outset—the antithesis of the creator in Genesis 1, whose creation is perfect and complete.

In Genesis 2–3, the tree of the knowledge of good and evil represents what Christian Science would consider the mistaken teaching that man is created from matter (dust and rib) and that matter has the ability to give life, pleasure, and power; that good is not the only power—evil is also a power; that men can be "as gods" in control of their lives (I Timothy 6:20–21 refers to this as false science). The Bible says this leads to death (I Corinthians 15:22: "For as in Adam all die, even so in Christ shall all be made alive"). The story of Adam and Eve breaks the first great commandment of Christianity, Judaism, and Islam—"Thou shalt have no other gods before me [Spirit]"—and illustrates how this belief in matter as a medium for creation or as a creative power mesmerizes thought and persuades people to believe that suffering is natural and death is inevitable.

Eddy found that if we believe that life and health are in matter and controlled by matter, then we also have to accept the belief that we are subject to disease, aging, accident, and death. If we doubt the existence of God or believe that He is not the only power and that there exist evil conditions or powers beyond God's power, this causes great fear, which results in suffering. She explains: "The procuring cause and foundation of all sickness is fear, ignorance, or sin. Disease is always induced by a false sense mentally entertained, not destroyed. Disease is an image of thought externalized. The mental state is called a material state. Whatever is cherished in mortal mind as the physical condition is imaged forth on the body" (1906, p. 411).

The word *sin* means "missing the mark" (Strong 1974), believing that anything can "overpower omnipotent and eternal Life" (Eddy 1906, pp. 428–29)—diverting one's life from God, Spirit, divine Love, through hatred, anger, dishonesty, self-indulgence, sexual license, or pagan worship of matter gods. Psalm 37 explains that when we keep our eyes focused on the mark, or goal, of "perfect man"—God's perfect creation—we find the presence of peace and the end of evil (Psalms 37:35–37). Psalm 138 continues, "The Lord will perfect that which concerns me." Jesus commanded, "Be ye therefore perfect even as your Father in heaven is perfect" (Matthew 5:48).

Resources for Living Well and for Healing

Eddy made a number of recommendations for students, followers, or practitioners of Christian Science. Foremost is obedience to the Ten Commandments, summed up in the two great commandments: "There is only one God; love God with all your heart, soul, strength, and mind"; and "Love your neighbor as yourself." In line with that, followers of Christian Science should avoid anything that interferes—drugs, alcohol, tobacco, caffeine, sensuality, and sex outside of marriage—with their ability to think clearly and follow God's guidance; live a balanced life; and begin each day with prayer and a study of a weekly Bible lesson which addresses many of the challenges people face each day.

A study of Eddy's textbook, *Science and Health*, has been sufficient to heal people of a wide variety of problems, such as rheumatism, tuberculosis, astigmatism, hernia, fibroid tumor, cataracts, valvular heart disease, cancer, Bright's disease, and pains of childbirth, to name a few (1906, pp. 600–700).

After people have studied her textbook and recognize its unique healing potential, they have the opportunity to take an intensive two-week Christian Science course called Primary Class Instruction, which is based on the chapter "Recapitulation" in *Science and Health*. During this course the students learn the fundamentals of Christian healing and how to give specific treatments through prayer for themselves and others. Teachers also discuss the ethics of Christian Science practice, including considerations that relate to confidentiality, availability, fees, and relationships with patients (for example, avoiding personal control, counseling, or involvement in personal affairs and avoiding mixing of spiritual and medical treatments).[3]

Although class instruction teaches people how to maintain their health, at times Christian Scientists face physical problems like anyone else. There are three provisions to support people seeking healing: (1) Christian Science practitioners are available to give treatment through prayer for people with any type of problem, including physical ones. (2) Christian Science nurses are available to care without medication for the physical needs of people dealing with injury, sickness, disease, mental problems, or aging. These services include private duty nurses; visiting nurse services; and camp and school nurses. (3) Christian Science nursing facilities staffed by Christian Science nurses are available for those requiring temporary care.

Students of Christian Science who want to advertise as Christian Science practitioners or nurses in the *Christian Science Journal* must meet certain requirements. Both practitioners and nurses must be members of the Mother Church and must have completed Primary Class Instruction with an authorized teacher of Christian Science.

Christian Science practitioners must have demonstrated an understanding of Christian Science in their own lives, based on deep study of the Bible and *Science and Health*. They must have an established, public practice with a record of success in healing; three references from patients who can attest to their healing work; full-time availability to answer calls (i.e., no other job); mentoring and recommendation from a Christian Science teacher or other experienced practitioner; and an interview with the Christian Science Publishing Society regarding the standards for an advertiser.

Christian Science nurses must have a "demonstrable knowledge of Christian Science practice," must "thoroughly understand the practical wisdom necessary in a sick room," and must be able to "take proper care of the sick" (Eddy 1908, p. 49). Preparation for Christian Science nursing includes courses and/or individual mentoring as well as a considerable period of supervised practice. This preparation generally takes between two and four years to complete and addresses the range of patients' needs, from those requiring light assistance to those needing full or extensive assistance, whether inpatient, outpatient, or in-home care.

The courses include, for example, skills required for preparing and modifying nourishment, and feeding the patient; assistance with lifting, moving, turning, and walking; the use of mobility aids; bed care and personal care; cleansing and bandaging skills; and responding to emergencies. Christian Science nursing is a spiritual and practical ministry that does not include medication but rather supports the patient's desire to rely solely on God for healing and provides compassionate care until the patient is again able to care for himself or herself.

Most Christian Science nursing facilities are relatively small, with 2 to 40 beds. There are about 26 facilities in the United States and others in Canada, Great Britain, Germany, and Switzerland. The majority of these facilities are designed to be short-term care facilities where individuals can find a refuge for prayer and healing. Many are Medicare providers. Individuals who are eligible for Medicare Part A and qualify as needing skilled care in a Religious Non-Medical Health Care Institution may apply for coverage while receiving care there.

The psychological atmosphere surrounding a patient is an important component of healing. Eddy counsels:

> The poor suffering heart needs its rightful nutriment, such as peace, patience in tribulation, and a priceless sense of the dear Father's loving-kindness. (1906, pp. 365–66)

> By conceding power to discord, a large majority of doctors depress mental energy, which is the only real recuperative power. Knowledge that we can accomplish the good we hope for, stimulates the system to act in the direction which Mind points out. The admission that any bodily condition is beyond the control of Mind disarms man, prevents him from helping himself, and enthrones matter through error. To those struggling with sickness, such admissions are discouraging—as much so as would be the advice to a man who is down in the world, that he should not try to rise above his difficulties. (1906, p. 394)

> Give sick people credit for sometimes knowing more than their doctors. Always support their trust in the power of Mind to sustain the body. Never tell the sick that they have more courage than strength. Tell them rather, that their strength is in proportion to their courage. (1906, p. 417)

Struggles of Believers with Contemporary Medical Practice

Eddy had great respect for doctors because they devote their lives to relieving suffering. She felt doctors would benefit from being students of Christian Science because this science would equip them with a "safe and sure medicine" (1906, p. 198; 1896, p. 252). In her chapter, "Science, Theology and Medicine," Eddy explains her understanding of true medicine: "God being All-in-all, He made medicine; but that medicine was Mind. It could not have been matter, which departs from the nature and character of Mind, God" (1906, p. 142).

Her objection was not to doctors but to matter-based medicine and treatments—a view of man as material and subject to sin, disease, and death, and a view of matter as more powerful than Spirit, God—contrary to Jesus's teaching and healing work. The fact that Jesus was sent as the Savior of the world and yet never used drugs or surgery but rather healed through prayer alone was one of the reasons she rejected material medicine. Jesus said, "It is the spirit who gives life; the flesh profits nothing" (John 6:63). He even turned people away from seeing him as the source of healing. He said, "I can of myself do nothing" (John 5:30, 19). "Why do you call me good? No one is good but one, that is, God. But if you want to enter into life, keep the commandments" (Matthew 19:17).

Matter-based medicine and treatments are constrained by their negative side-effects, high cost, and inaccessibility to large numbers around the world; and yet the Bible promises that God's gifts bring only good, not suffering, and that they bless everyone—no one is excluded (James 1:17). As Eddy writes, "In divine Science, where prayers are mental, *all* may avail themselves of God as 'a very present help in trouble'" (1906, pp. 12–13).

Christian Scientists are free to choose whatever form of treatment they feel works best for them, but generally speaking they choose an entirely spiritual approach to all forms of suffering or malfunction because they find it so effective and reliable. The Mother Church (the organizing body of Christian Science which is governed by its church manual) does not dictate the personal choices of health care for its members—for example, whether or not to have surgery. In fact, Eddy makes a provision for a Christian Scientist to have bones set by surgery:

> Until the advancing age admits the efficacy and supremacy of Mind, it is better for Christian Scientists to leave surgery and the adjustment of broken bones and dislocations to the fingers of a surgeon, while the mental healer confines himself chiefly to mental reconstruction and to the prevention of inflammation. Christian Science is always the most skilful surgeon, but surgery is the branch of its healing which will be last acknowledged. However, it is but just to say that the author has already in her possession well-authenticated records of the cure, by herself and her students through mental surgery alone, of broken bones, dislocated joints, and spinal vertebrae. (1906, p. 401)

Eddy also made provision for Christian Science practitioners to consult with medical doctors in certain cases (1908, p. 47), and there may be times when Christian Science nurses need to consult with doctors. If a patient has received medical treatment before seeking healing through spiritual reliance, or chooses to seek medical assistance after entering a Christian Science facility, a Christian Science nurse might communicate (within HIPAA regulations) with medical personnel regarding the care. For example, a patient who has chosen to have an X ray and a bone set, or surgery, and is requiring skilled assistance with continued care might request to have this care without medication and with the support of Christian Science nursing. The Christian Science nurse would need to consider appropriate activities for the patient and skilled care regarding mobility and other matters.

I received a call from a hospital chaplain who said she was working with a Christian Scientist who had been diagnosed with an advanced case of cancer. The patient was trying to decide between medical and Christian Science treatment, but he was overwhelmed with fear, pain, and a feeling of having been abandoned by God. I shared some passages from the Bible with the chaplain that she could read to the patient to comfort and support him as he prayed about which course to take. The chaplain found the passages helpful and was happy to read them to the patient. She also took the name of some Christian Science practitioners to contact.

The best support a doctor or nurse can give to a Christian Scientist who has been brought to a hospital but wants Christian Science treatment is to help the person find a Bible, a copy of *Science and Health*, and a Christian Science practitioner so he or she can pray about what step to take or choice to make. Christian Science is the science of God's tender, loving care for each of us.

Although Eddy makes provision for practitioners to consult with a medical doctor, she is also clear that the medicine of Mind and the medicine of matter tend to negate each other because Spirit and matter are opposites. The Bible explains: "To be carnally minded is death; but to be spiritually minded is life and peace. Because the carnal mind is enmity against God: for it is not subject to the law of God, neither indeed can be" (Romans 8:6–7).

It would be unethical, Eddy says, for a Christian Scientist to give treatment to someone who makes a conscious decision to rely on medical treatment because Christian Science treatment affirms the powerlessness of matter and would undermine the patient's choice of treatment. In like manner, when a patient chooses to rely on Christian Science treatment, medical diagnoses, prognoses, and treatments tend to undermine the patient's ability to put all his confidence in God.

My family has relied exclusively on Christian Science treatment for four generations and has found God, the divine Mind, to be the most effective physician and surgeon. When my uncle was a young man in the Air Force, he was diagnosed with spinal meningitis. The medical treatment failed, and he went into a coma. The doctors told my grandmother there was nothing more they could do for him and they doubted he would survive. However, after five days of Christian Science treatment he came out of the coma. He was soon completely healed, returned to training and became a pilot.

My father was told by a friend who was a surgeon that the lump on my father's forehead was a tumor requiring immediate surgery; however, my father healed it through prayer alone. Both my brother and my cousin were in serious car accidents with multiple broken bones, and both were healed through prayer alone.

In my cousin's case, he was taken to the hospital and given drugs before my aunt arrived. The doctors feared he would not survive because of the negative reaction he had to the drugs and the severity of the injuries. Through prayer, that prognosis was turned around, and he began recovering. Because my uncle was not yet a Christian Scientist, my aunt let him choose between medical or Christian Science treatment for their son. The doctors said it would be six months before my cousin could walk again. My uncle chose to rely exclusively on Christian Science treatment, affirming that his son was governed by the law of God, Spirit, which maintains our life and health, and not by so-called laws of chance, accident, or physiology. Eight weeks later, my cousin went on a 50-mile hike with his Boy Scout troop completely healed. Later he joined the Navy and was declared fit by the medical examiner.

My cousin's healing took place many years ago, when doctors and hospitals were more supportive of patients' decisions about their own health care. However, in the last couple of decades, that interaction between doctors and patients, including respect for patients' rights and choices, seems rare. Often Christian Scientists or those turning to Christian Science after first seeking medical help have raised the concern that once a person is in the medical system, it is difficult to get out again if they so desire.[4]

Challenging and Reinforcing Contemporary Medical Practice

A significant body of medical writing questions the growing medicalization of the human condition (e.g., the medicalization of childbirth or the "epidemic of obesity"). It points to the mental nature of suffering and challenges the medical tendency to reduce everything to matter and the brain (Crabtree 1993; Kelly et al. 2007). Although this literature cannot be said to prove the effectiveness of prayer to heal, it nevertheless suggests a relationship between prayer and healing which cannot be ignored.

For example, the authors of *Irreducible Mind* write: "The hypothesis that consciousness is the product of brain processes, or that mind is merely the subjective concomitant of neurological events, has been and remains the almost universal assumption in neuroscience and psychology. Investigations of certain extraordinary circumstances, however, reveal phenomena that call into question this assumption" (Kelly et al. 2007, p. 367). In discussing the genesis of their book, Kelly and coauthors state: "By the year 2000 our discussions had advanced to the point where we believed we could demonstrate, empirically, that the materialistic consensus which undergirds practically all of current mainstream psychology, neuroscience, and philosophy of mind is fundamentally flawed. . . . In a nutshell, we are arguing for abandonment of the current materialistic synthesis, and for the restoration of causally efficacious conscious mental life to its proper place at the center of our science" (2007, pp. xiii–xiv).

The teachings of Christian Science can seem hard to accept when the five physical senses confirm in no uncertain terms that a bone is broken, or that disease is spreading, or that a person has died. And yet for years a wide variety of medical studies has questioned the reliability of the physical senses. Studies of the placebo effect (evident when people think they are receiving a drug or treatment and improve even though they were given no drug or treatment) and of the nocebo effect (seen when people think they have been exposed to a disease or something noxious in the air, and then develop the symptoms, suffer, perhaps even die, without being exposed to any disease) are examples of this. They illustrate the mental nature of all suffering.

A striking example of this is the case of a group of patients diagnosed with angina pectoris, who were offered surgery (ligation of the internal mammary artery) in the hopes of improving their heart condition (Dimond, Kittle, and Crockett 1960). Five of 18 patients—which 5 was not known either by the patients or by their cardiologists—received sham rather than real surgery (a slit in their chest which was then sewn up again) and experienced improvement comparable to that of patients who underwent real surgery. In fact, all 5 reported improvement ranging from feeling much better to being cured, whereas

4 of the 13 who actually did undergo surgery were disappointed with the improvement or got worse. This 1960 study is cited because it is unique and because, given ethical concerns, it will never be repeated now that there is successful coronary intervention technology. It does add to the growing body of evidence regarding placebo (faith-based) effects.

A recent issue of *Scientific American Mind* (Niemi 2009) described a man who was dying of cancer of the lymph nodes, with orange-size tumors in his neck, groin, chest, and abdomen. Doctors had exhausted all available treatments. But "Mr. Wright," the patient, was confident that a new anticancer drug called Krebiozen would cure him. Although he was "bedridden and fighting for each breath" when he received his first injection, within three days his tumors had shrunk by half, and after 10 more days of treatment, he was discharged from the hospital. However, two months later, on reading reports that Krebiozen was worthless, he died within two days.

There are many examples of the power of hypnotism to make people believe they are physically suffering when it is simply the power of suggestion (Kelly et al. 2007, pp. 179–239). Kelly and associates point out: "Hypnotic suggestion *properly administered to suitable subjects* can bring about psychobiological changes in the total organism which are impossible of attainment in the waking state" (2007, p. 182). Sorcery, which is practiced extensively in Africa and countries with African descendants, is a clear example of this. Its practitioners explain that when a sorcerer or witch doctor puts a curse on a person (saying that the individual will suffer an accident, a disease, or death), it happens just as they say it will. This practice evolved out of a centuries-old belief that there is a spiritual side of material life and a belief in the power of thought to control things in the material world—mixing good and evil in practice.

Voodoo or hex death is found not just in folk societies but also in Western cultures: "The belief that one is going to die may be generated, not by a witch doctor's curse, but by . . . a doctor's pronouncement of a hopeless condition . . . , or some other suggestion accepted by the patient" (Kelly et al. 2007, p. 125; see also Eddy 1906, pp. 197–98). Eddy explains: "Mortal existence is a dream of pain and pleasure in matter, a dream of sin, sickness, and death; and it is like the dream we have in sleep, in which every one recognizes his condition to be wholly a state of mind. In both the waking and the sleeping dream, the dreamer thinks that his body is material and the suffering is in that body" (Eddy 1906, p. 188).[5]

Once people have studied Christian Science, learned the omnipotence of good and the powerlessness of sorcery, a curse has no effect on them, and the disease, suffering, or danger disappears.[6] However, it is important to point out that this is not an intellectual, mystical, or ritual exercise. It is the power of divine Love expressed in unselfishness, patience, tenderness, compassion, and forgiveness—found in obedience to the two great commandments and in Jesus's Sermon on the Mount, discussed earlier—which overcomes fear, and fully and finally reduces sorcery to its powerlessness. Believing that there are two powers—good and evil—undermines one's ability to overcome evil. Only by understanding that Spirit is good alone, and is the only power, can one overcome fear and suffering. St. John said, "There is no fear in love; but perfect love casts out fear because fear involves torment" (I John 4:18).

Kelly and his coauthors point to many medically documented cases of healing through faith or prayer of even potentially fatal diseases that failed to respond to medical treatment (2007, pp. 130–39). The Christian Science Church has had magazines since 1883, and now Web sites, that regularly document healings through Christian Science treatment, including many examples where there has been a medical diagnosis.[7]

For example, over the period from 1969 to 1988, the *Christian Science Journal* and *Christian Science Sentinel* printed more than 7,100 testimonies of physical healing. Of these, 2,228 involved medically diagnosed conditions; 2,400 were healings of children, more than 600 of which had been medically diagnosed. These children's cases included "spinal meningitis (in several cases after antibiotics failed to help), pneumonia and double pneumonia, diabetes, food poisoning, heart disorders, loss of eyesight from chemical burns, pleurisy, stomach obstruction, epilepsy, goiter, leukemia, malaria, mastoiditis, polio, rheumatic fever, and ruptured appendix" (Christian Science Board of Directors 1989, p. 68; see also Christian Science Publishing 1966).

While some medical practitioners are open to the idea that prayer could effect physiological change and that suffering could be mental, many are not open to anything but a material view of life and healing. Christian Scientists and many others are troubled by (1) the lack of freedom of choice experienced by many people in relation to medicine, including legal pressure put on parents to choose medical over spiritual means (even when medicine admits its lack of certainty or its danger); and (2) the prevailing tendency to see disease as the natural and inevitable state of mankind, manifested in an aggressive diagnosing or looking for disease, even in healthy people. My perception is that before the 1980s in the United States, it was easier to practice Christian Science treatment without interference.

Perhaps one of the reasons that Christian Science healing was so effective and widespread in the United States during the first century after Eddy shared her findings was the U.S. tradition of democracy and respect for religious freedom (together with a deep love of the Bible and a strong Christian foundation focused on only one God). Fear of persecution and penalties for choosing prayer have at times inhibited healing through prayer.

Eddy points out that both the doctor's thought and the patient's thought are important for healing: "A patient's belief is more or less moulded and formed by his doctor's belief in the case, even though the doctor says nothing to support his theory. His thoughts and his patient's commingle, and the stronger thoughts rule the weaker. Hence the importance that doctors be Christian Scientists" (Eddy 1906, p. 198). Negative mental states on the doctor's part, such as impatience, irritation, anger, indifference, fear, or hopelessness, directly affect patients' thoughts and expectations, as we saw in the medical studies reviewed by Kelly and others in *Irreducible Mind*.

Christian Science and Culture

Western culture and medicine tend to see everything as material and therefore appear more antagonistic toward the belief in the spiritual and more likely to restrict the free practice of healing through prayer. Asian and African cultures, on the other hand, are open to the idea of the spiritual and mental nature of things in the human experience and are thus more open to considering nonallopathic methods of healing, including prayer. To the degree that a culture respects freedom of religion and recognizes the power of one God, Spirit, who creates only good, to that degree healing thrives.

Over the last couple of decades, a culture of fear—of seeing danger in every direction—appears to be developing in society and undermining people's recognition that health is natural to all of us. And yet the Bible assures us, "God has not given us the spirit of fear; but of power, and of love, and of a sound mind" (II Timothy 1:7).

The U.S. culture places emphasis on the body—fearing it, worshipping it—and one often hears, "Listen to your body." This is contrary to the biblical foundation of Christian Science healing, which teaches us to silence the body or physical senses. The Bible says, "Be silent, O all flesh before the Lord" (Zechariah 2:13); we need "to be absent from the body, and to be present with the Lord" (II Corinthians 5:8) if we want to maintain our health. Although disciplining thought and not listening to the body have always been natural to athletes who succeed in breaking limitations, today our culture tends to undermine this mental discipline.

In the past few decades, Western medical culture, particularly in the United States, has questioned the use of prayer in children's cases, and yet the single thing I am most grateful for on the part of my parents is that when I was a child they handled all physical problems through prayer in Christian Science and taught me from my youngest years to turn to God in prayer. My healings were quick and painless. And even better, I have found Christian Science to be the best preventive medicine. My brother, sister, and I all found as children that Christian Science treatment freed us from fear, limitations, and many childhood problems. Now our grown children have chosen this form of health care and have found consistent health and well-being.

Christian Science parents naturally love their children and want them to thrive. The Bible repeatedly stresses that it is never God's will that children or anyone else die (Ezekiel 18:23; Psalms 103:2–4). God's will is that we prosper and be healthy. Like any good parent, Christian Science parents want to choose the form of treatment that is most effective, reliable, and immediate, and that is why they choose Christian Science prayer so often. A growing number of parents today, including some doctors, question the safety of inoculations for children.[8] Christian Scientists, generally speaking, do not give their children inoculations because they have found a safer, more effective way of preventing disease, and that is daily prayer for their children—prayer based on the Science of the Christ.

Addressing and Accessing Spirituality in Practice

Prayer in Christian Science affirms the allness and supremacy of God, Spirit, and the consequent powerlessness and nothingness of evil in any form. As a practitioner, I am striving to lift my thought and the thought of my patient up to the Christ—the divine understanding of perfect God, perfect man (Eddy 1906, p. 259). This means sometimes specifically addressing, through prayer, any fear, ignorance, or sin in the thought of the patient. Other times, both the patient and the practitioner so fully understand man's inseparability from

God, man's true nature as God's perfect reflection, and the allness of God, Spirit, and consequent powerlessness of matter that the healing comes quickly and naturally.

Christian Scientists never ignore a physical problem; rather, they choose the form of treatment they have found to be most immediate and reliable with no negative side effects—the medicine of Mind. For example, one night around 3:00 a.m., I received a call from a man whose wife appeared to have just died. She had had a heart attack and stopped breathing. He tried to revive her but could not, so he called an ambulance. Then he called me.

I asked him to put the phone to her ear, and I spoke to her: "You know that God is your life and that you can never be separated from God. You know that God is the only Mind and nothing can keep you from hearing God's healing message." Then I put down the phone and continued praying. In the morning they called back to say she revived immediately after I spoke to her and felt fine. She later learned from a doctor that excessive caffeine and taking energy supplements containing ephedrine can have this effect on the body (she had previously had heart murmurs). She realized that although she had never taken medication of any sort, she had believed her strength and alertness depended on material supplements rather than God (Isaiah 40:31). She stopped relying on those things and has not had a recurrence of the heart problem.

The question is often asked, why Christian Science treatment cannot be tested by controlled clinical studies. The Bible explains that "eye hath not seen nor ear heard, neither have entered in to the heart of man, the things which God hath prepared for them that love him" (I Corinthians 2:9). Health is entirely and exclusively a spiritual state. It cannot be measured by the limited ability of the physical senses. These senses know only disease and deterioration; they cannot even recognize health. Paul said we live, move, and have our being in Spirit (Acts 17:28). Spiritual sense alone communicates health.

Conclusion

Christian Science offers healers and patients, regardless of religious background, a perspective and an approach to healing that has proven to be effective and reliable for over a century. The apostle Paul summed up the truth of the complete system of healing in Christian Science (Eddy 1913, p. 113) in two verses in the Bible, Romans 8:1–2: "There is therefore now no condemnation [which has as one of its meanings "incurability"] to those who are in Christ

Jesus, who do not walk according to the flesh, but according to the Spirit. For the law of the Spirit of life in Christ Jesus has made me free from the law of sin and death."

Eddy taught that "when the Science of being is universally understood, every man will be his own physician, and Truth will be the universal panacea" (Eddy 1906, p. 144).

NOTES

1. The Hebrew, Christian, and Muslim Scriptures all contain references to the Messiah, Savior, or Christ and the power to heal disease, injury, blindness, deafness, and insanity through spiritual means alone. Examples in the Hebrew Bible include Daniel 3; Exodus 3–4; I Kings 19; I Kings 17:17–24; II Kings 4:17–37; Psalms 103:2–4. The birth story of Jesus appears in the Quran 3:42–51. See also, Eddy 1906, p. 328.

2. See note 1. The Christian Scriptures were written in Aramaic and Greek, and the Jewish Scriptures in Hebrew. Depending on the translator and the language, a text may read "knowledge" or "science," because both are accurate translations. The French translation, for example, uses "science": "the science of God" (Romans 11:33); "God's science is perfect" (Job 37:16); "the fear [respect] of God, Spirit, is the beginning of science" (Proverbs 1:7); "in Christ are found all the treasures of wisdom and science" (Colossians 2:2–3); Paul warns against "false science which turns people away from faith in God" (I Timothy 6: 20–21). Quotations translated from Second 1910.

3. For more on the ethics of Christian Science practice and nursing, see the following. On ethics as defined in Jesus's Sermon on the Mount (Matt. 5–7), Eddy 1906, pp. 444:31–446:4; 144:14-22; and 145:16. And from Eddy 1908, on ethics, 40:5; 83:4, 11; 84:18; on practice, 46:12–47:10; 82:16; 92:3–11; on nursing, 49:7–16. For more on surgery and vaccinations, see Eddy 1896, p. 243; Eddy 1913, pp. 344–45.

4. An interesting question arose while I was in law school about how much control one organization should be given over an individual's choice of health care. I took a course on antitrust and hospital law, in which the professor expressed his concern about the control the AMA appeared to have over all health care practices and the ability to restrict which ones could be practiced, explaining that such a control violates antitrust law, but that the public and the government were reluctant to challenge them.

5. For more on the effect of doctors' and/or patients' beliefs on the patient's physical condition, see Kelly et al. 2007, pp. 123–27, specifically the following: P. 123: "Hopelessness . . . correlated with higher rates of death from cardiovascular disease, cancer, and violence or injury. . . . Association between depression or hopelessness and cancer . . . or cardiovascular disease." P. 127: The case of an elderly man who died after being given the diagnosis of widespread incurable liver cancer (which he believed); but an autopsy revealed the diagnosis was false. P. 130: "Religious involvement correlates with improved immune system function and a lower risk of cardiovascular disease, hypertension, stroke, pain, and mortality in general." P. 131: "In 42 independent studies based on a sample of almost 126,000 people, the meta-analysis also revealed a significant correlation between religious involvement and reduction of mortality from a variety of causes." Pp. 221–24: Medical studies talk about "maternal impressions" in which a

mother is mesmerized (greatly impressed and frightened) by pictures of deformity, for example, and then her newborn child manifests the deformity. See also Eddy 1906, p. 178.

6. As manager of the international Christian Science Board of Lectureship, I was responsible for training our lecturers in Africa, who are all Christian Science practitioners. They each had examples of the harmful effect that sorcery seems to have, even on educated people, but each gave specific examples of how the belief in sorcery lost all power to harm them once they studied Christian Science and realized that God, good, is the only Mind governing us and never causes suffering or death.

7. The following weekly, monthly, or quarterly publications by the First Church of Christ, Scientist, along with their Web sites, document healings through Christian Science treatment, including conditions that have been medically diagnosed: the *Christian Science Journal*, the *Christian Science Sentinel* (both accessible on the Web at www.spirituality.com), and the *Herald of Christian Science* (printed in 14 languages and posted in 22 languages on the Web site, www.csherald.com); also see www.christian science.com.

8. As an attorney in the Legal and Legislative Department of our Committee on Publication at the Mother Church, I received several calls from medical doctors asking if they could use our legal provisions to protect their children from having to receive inoculations. They said they gave inoculations to their patients because the patients wanted them, but the doctors did not feel they were safe for their own children.

REFERENCES

Christian Science Publishing 1966. *A Century of Christian Science Healing*. Boston. Christian Science Publishing Society.

Christian Science Board of Directors. 1989. *Freedom and Responsibility: Christian Science Healing for Children*. Boston: First Church of Christ, Scientist.

Crabtree, A. 1993. *From Mesmer to Freud: Magnetic Sleep and the Roots of Psychological Healing*. New Haven: Yale University Press.

Dimond, E. G., C. F. Kittle, and J. E. Crockett. 1960. Comparison of internal mammary artery ligation and sham operation for angina pectoris. *American Journal of Cardiology* 5:483–86.

Eddy, M. B. 1892. *Retrospection and Introspection*. Boston: First Church of Christ, Scientist.

———. 1896. *Miscellaneous Writings, 1883–1896*. Boston: First Church of Christ, Scientist.

———. 1906. *Science and Health with Key to the Scriptures*. Boston: First Church of Christ, Scientist.

———. 1908. *Church Manual of the First Church of Christ, Scientist in Boston, Massachusetts*. Boston: First Church of Christ, Scientist.

———. 1913. *The First Church of Christ, Scientist and Miscellany*. Boston: First Church of Christ, Scientist.

Kelly, E. F., E. W. Kelly, A. Crabtree, A. Gauld, M. Grosso, and B. Greyson. 2007. *Irreducible Mind: Toward a Psychology for the Twenty-first Century*. Lanham, MD: Rowman and Littlefield.

Kohlenberger, J. R., III, general editor. 2004. *The Essential Evangelical Parallel Bible: New King James Version of the Bible*. New York: Oxford University Press.

Niemi, B. 2009. Cure in the mind. *Scientific American Mind*, Feb.–Mar., pp. 42–49.
Second, L., trans. 1910. *La Bible et Parole Vivante*. Grezieu la Varenne: Association Viens et Vois.
Strong, J. 1974. *Strong's Exhaustive Concordance*. Nashville: Abingdon Press.
Wolf, S. 1950. Effects of suggestion and conditioning on the action of chemical agents in human subjects: The pharmacology of placebos. *Journal of Clinical Investigation* 29:100–109.

CHAPTER TEN

Jehovah's Witnesses

Jon Schiller, M.D.

Few religious groups have proved as disquieting to contemporary society as Jehovah's Witnesses. There are a number of paradoxes:

- Although they are recognized as a law-abiding and peace-loving people, Witnesses have over the past century found themselves imprisoned for their convictions in virtually every part of the world.
- Though biblical beliefs permeate their approach to life, they hold that religions, often under the guise of spiritual motivation, have proved a negative force in the world.
- Known generally for a strong moral standard and a high regard for family life, they are accused of allowing family members to die rather than accept blood transfusions.

To address the challenges Jehovah's Witnesses present to the medical community, we need to examine what motivates Jehovah's Witnesses to think and behave as they do. This chapter will consider three questions:

1. Who are Jehovah's Witnesses?
2. How best can we face the singular challenge they present to the medical community?
3. What are some spiritual implications for the practicing clinician?

Who Are Jehovah's Witnesses?

For that matter, who is Jehovah? Jehovah's Witnesses identify *Jehovah* as the personal name of God. For them, this is not a small point, as they believe they can show multiple instances where that name has been expunged from Bible translations (one of the few left in some renditions being *hallelujah*, or "praise to Jah"). For them, God, Jehovah, is not a trinity, but the sole creator, the all-powerful Father; and Jesus Christ is his only-begotten, firstborn son. With this background, for our purposes we could group the beliefs of Jehovah's Witnesses into four main teachings. (The Jehovah's Witness Web site, watchtower.org, discusses beliefs in much more detail.)

1. *Death is the opposite of life.* For the Jehovah's Witness, when a person dies, he is dead, out of existence, and not living on somewhere in some other state of being. There is no immortal soul that leaves the body; there is certainly no fear of eternal torment in a hellfire. With this belief, Witnesses place a high value on life here on this earth and a high value on taking care of their personal health. The hope for the future of a dead person is for a resurrection through the ransom sacrifice of Jesus—a resurrection back to perfect health on a paradise earth as God originally intended. Witnesses are thus led to have a pragmatic view toward end-of-life matters, not expecting divine intervention or miraculous cures on their behalf. Nor do they believe in intercessory healing prayers. Though there were miraculous healings in the first century by Jesus and the apostles, Witnesses teach that these healings served the purpose of dramatizing Jehovah's approval of the fledgling Christian congregation. "Once mature or fully established, rather than pointing to special gifts, the Christian congregation would point to its display of unswerving faith, hope, and love as evidence of God's approval" (Watchtower Society 2009, p. 28).

2. *The future worldview is optimistic.* Witnesses believe in a positive hope for the future of mankind on earth, after the coming battle between the forces of good and evil, in the battle the Bible calls Armageddon. They believe this will be accomplished by means of a new government, a world government under Christ which in reality Christians have prayed for over the centuries: "Thy kingdom come, thy will be done, on earth as it is in heaven." For now, the explanation for the bad things that happen lies in a combination of factors. In our imperfection, we humans tend to make poor decisions. Furthermore, this world is temporarily under the power of rebellious spirit creatures, who are the

main force behind the death, pain, and evil on the earth today. Evil may find its way to any of us, good or bad, in the present world, but it may be endured with prayer. By this frequent communication through Jesus with the Father, Jehovah, the Witness maintains a close spiritual relationship that provides endurance for the trials that must come. Thus, although a Jehovah's Witnesses would, in public and private, pray for someone who is ill, the prayer would not be for a special cure, but instead for wisdom, endurance, and integrity under trail. The Witness would also try to accompany that prayer with practical, helpful assistance to the sick one.

3. *Christians today should be a worldwide family, living in peace.* Until the battle of Armageddon, Witnesses feel it important to stay neutral in the politics and wars of this system. Because Jesus before his death stated, "My kingdom is no part of this world," they feel impelled to stay strictly aloof from the nationalistic wars and political issues that divide peoples. They feel that not only are all races and societies equal in the eyes of God, but that the Witness "family" extends worldwide without respect for manmade national boundaries, so that to participate in or support any of the world's conflicts would be in essence fighting against their own brothers and sisters in other parts of the world. Refusing to be any part of armed conflict, Witnesses in Germany in World War II were sent to concentration camps and killed. In her book, *The Nazi State and the New Religions*, Christine E. King notes that "one out of every two German Witnesses was imprisoned, one in four lost their lives." Yet, "against all odds, Witnesses in the camps met and prayed together, produced literature and made converts. Sustained by their friendship, and, unlike many other prisoners, well aware of the reasons why such places existed and why they should suffer thus, Witnesses proved a small but memorable band of prisoners, marked by the violet triangle and noted for their courage and their convictions" (King 1982, p. 158). They were also incarcerated during the war in the Western countries (the United States, Great Britain, France, and elsewhere) for the same reasons. Today in many countries—South Korea, Argentina, Armenia, and Eritrea, among others—young Witnesses are now in prison for refusal to be part of the military (Watchtower Society 2008). However, Witnesses believe that in their organization they have achieved earthwide the peace that the world dreams of, and they are enthusiastic about promulgating this teaching in any way open to them, even door-to-door where possible.

4. *The Bible is the true guide for living.* Finally, and critically for our discussion, Jehovah's Witnesses believe that real happiness, both now and in the fu-

ture, comes from closely following the direction of God as set down in scripture and especially as taught by the greatest teacher on earth, Jesus Christ. Witnesses believe not only that scriptural direction is timeless and infallible, but also that closely following it will make them better husbands, wives, and children and will offer a sure hope for the future. Thus, their beliefs have a strong tone of morality and of caring for their bodies (for example, they neither use tobacco nor abuse alcohol), and spiritual values permeate their lives. As a group they have the reputation of knowing their Bible well, for to them it is not just the "Good Book," but the daily guide to life. Spirituality is a thing that requires constant vigilance and effort because of the draining effect of the materialism, violence, and immorality of contemporary society. The promise of Jesus is that, if they just do their best to be faithful, even if they die, they will be resurrected.

In discussions with medical personnel regarding Jehovah's Witnesses, the question often arises, "What are the repercussions to a Witness who decides to take a blood transfusion?" There is no overall rule, and each case, while infrequent, would be considered individually. As outlined above, Jehovah's Witnesses follow a biblical moral code, and they are protective of their reputation for adhering to it. Thus, a person who decided to cheat on his taxes, for example, could not be one of Jehovah's Witnesses. The same principle holds with regard to adultery, stealing, or, for that matter, accepting blood transfusions. A person can make a mistake in one of these issues and be forgiven, but if one knowingly flouts any of these standards, that person simply is not one of Jehovah's Witnesses.

In summary, by following scriptural principles—by learning to get along, by not judging others, by combating evil thoughts and immoral inclinations—Jehovah's Witnesses firmly believe they will benefit now and everlastingly. (See Watchtower Society 2007.)

Challenge to the Medical Community

The medical community is becoming increasingly cognizant of Jehovah's Witnesses. For instance, the journal *Trauma* reports that "as the most rapidly growing religious group in the western world, Jehovah's Witnesses represent an international religious organization comprised of more than 6.7 million members worldwide, with more than one million members in the United States" (Hughes,

Ullery, and Barie 2008, p. 273). Likewise, *Marrow Transplantation* notes, "Through aggressive evangelism and missionary work, they have emerged as a major worldwide religious group" (Sloan and Ballen 2008, p. 837).

To Jehovah's Witnesses, one of the biblical commandments, no more or no less important than the other Bible commands, is to abstain from blood. They hold that scripturally, the life is in the blood and is sacred to God. Blood is not to be "spilled" or "eaten," according to the Bible (Genesis 9:4; Acts 15:28, 29). Thus, though there may be temporary gains from winning a war or taking a blood transfusion, ultimately the real hope is in the new world government made possible by the ransom provision of the blood of Jesus (Watchtower Society 1990). That is where Witnesses place their faith for a better future. Incidentally, by keeping these convictions, they do not feel that God is withholding something beneficial from them, as we shall see.

In the 1940s and 1950s, when they first reasoned that transfusing blood was equivalent to eating it, they were seen as "odd" and misguided. By the '60s and early '70s, accusations became more serious as a result of inflammatory reporting of occasional adverse results attributed to Witnesses' stubborn refusal to accept blood transfusions. In those days everyone knew that anemia below 10 g/dl hemoglobin was life threatening and needed to be treated with transfusion, and quickly. Many surgical procedures could not even be attempted without resort to transfusion. Downside? There was no downside to speak of with blood transfusions. The blood supply was certainly safe; everyone knew that. Witnesses were sometimes labeled fanatics at best, lunatics at worst, who were denying themselves surgeries and optimal medical care for lack of the "gift of life," blood transfusions.

Then, in the 1970s and 1980s, three things happened that changed the situation. First, a deluge of articles began to appear in the medical literature demonstrating that the medical approach to anemia needed adjustment and that the human body could tolerate much lower hemoglobin levels than previously thought. Concomitantly, the surgical literature published case reports and review articles which ultimately demonstrated that, if properly approached, virtually any surgery could be done safely on Jehovah's Witnesses.

A second major development involved an initiative on the part of the Watchtower Society, a legal designation of Jehovah's Witnesses. Reasoning that much of the adverse publicity was due to miscommunication and misunderstanding, and that the result was deleterious to both the medical community and the Witnesses, the society mounted a major effort to reach out to doctors and hospitals around the world. Further, there was education within the organization as to what the individual Witness could do to avoid confrontation. Hospital liaison committees were established, and these were available when called on by doctors or hospitals to help resolve problems.

Then came the third development. AIDS was first recognized by the U.S. Centers for Disease Control and Prevention in 1981 and its cause, HIV, identified in the early 1980s. Soon the enormous impact of this new scourge became clear, along with the fact that it could be transmitted in blood transfusions.

As a result of all this, Jehovah's Witnesses no longer seemed so crazy, and they too felt some vindication that God had in fact not been withholding something good from them.

In the years since then, much progress has been made in the relations between Jehovah's Witnesses and the medical community. First, there is the growth in the study of bloodless surgery and medicine. In addition, Witnesses are reputed to be good patients. They take care of their health, pay their bills, are honest, and believe in science, medication, and surgery. For religious reasons, they prefer nonblood alternatives, which are now readily available worldwide. Putney reports that "more than 100 bloodless medicine and surgery centers currently exist in the United States, and this number will surely increase" (Putney 2007, p. 264). Worldwide, the best estimate is that there are about 350 bloodless centers (Watchtower Society, personal communication). There is also an international database of hospitals providing blood-conserving services, the Society for the Advancement of Blood Management (Pasci 2008).

The question arises, why such a burgeoning worldwide effort in this field? Surely this is not all just because of Jehovah's Witnesses. It turns out that many medical economists and clinicians are examining this issue.

In addition to the expense and difficulty in obtaining adequate blood supplies, more research is examining the downside of blood usage. According to Putney (2007, p. 263), "Some of these risks, such as an increased surgical infection rate are well documented by research. . . . Other risks, such as the possible transmission of infectious prions, . . . we are only beginning to understand." There are also the non-infectious hazards of transfusion: incompatibility and mistransfusion, transfusion-related acute lung injury (TRALI), and cardiopulmonary toxicity, to name a few. Especially intriguing is the growing body of evidence regarding immune effects. Notes a Brazilian pediatric intensivist: "One of the least considered but significant effects of transfusion is immunosuppression which also contributes to mortality. . . . studies have demonstrated that blood transfusions have been associated to higher incidences of postoperative infections in several populations, and greater rates of neoplasia recurrence according to the number of transfusions done" (Digieri et al. 2006, p. 190).

Furthermore, the literature regarding the body's tolerance of anemia has recently become more illuminating, thus putting into question the need for transfusion in many cases. Hughes and associates report: "Considering the rarity with which Jehovah's Witnesses die from severe anemia after major elective surgery and that transfusion may actually portend a worse prognosis, Carson et al. explored the clinical consequences of low hemoglobin concentration in individuals who decline blood transfusion for religious reasons. . . . it was evident that morbidity and mortality rates dramatically increased only when the hemoglobin concentration decreased below 5 g/dl" (Hughes, Ullery, and Barie 2008, p. 241). And according to the same article, other researchers cite an even lower hemoglobin level: "The 'terminal hemoglobin threshold' may be as low as 3 g/dl to 5 g/dl in some patients, and transfusion alone is not without potential deleterious physiologic effects" (p. 245). An article in the *American Journal of Medicine* says, "There are also case reports of JW patients who have survived very low blood counts, dipping as low as 1.5 gm/dl, before erythropoiesis resumes" (Remmers and Speer 2006, p. 1015). Most experts now recommend using no specific number as a "trigger" for transfusion, but instead carefully monitoring the hemodynamic stability of the individual patient (Digieri et al. 2006; Remmers and Speer 2006).

As a result of the application of these principles, one finds these statements in the recent literature:

> The goal of this case report is to alert doctors about the several inherent risks of blood transfusions and provide alternative tools for treating severe anemia, especially in critically ill children without using blood products. (Digieri et al. 2006, p. 191)

> In 2003, Varela et al. conducted a retrospective cohort study of 556 patients comparing the risks of death after major trauma for Jehovah's Witnesses and other religious groups (i.e., Catholics, Baptists, and others). . . . Varela et al. concluded that Jehovah's Witnesses had no increased risk of death after major trauma compared with other religious groups. . . . In addition to the apparent lack of mortality benefit attributable to transfusion, recent data suggest that Jehovah's Witnesses may actually benefit with regard to improved clinical outcomes from the decision to forego transfusion. (Hughes, Ullery, and Barie 2008, p. 240)

> One thing is clear: strategies to reduce blood loss benefit patients. Many transfusions can be avoided simply by taking every precaution to minimize blood loss. . . . Reducing or eliminating blood transfusions also results in improved patient outcomes. Many studies document an increase in morbidity and mortality after a blood transfusion. (Putney 2007, p. 264)

These positive results with blood-conserving approaches have been reported worldwide across the medical specialties: obstetrics (Massiah et al. 2007, for Scotland), spinal surgery (Joseph et al. 2008, for the United States), head and neck surgery (Adelola, Ahmed, and Fenton 2008, for Ireland), liver transplantation (Jeffrey et al. 2007, for Australia), cardiac surgery (Casati et al. 2007, for Italy), and even bone marrow transplantation (Sloan and Ballen 2008, for the United States). (Jehovah's Witnesses as an organization does not proscribe transplants, though some Witnesses may not accept them [Watchtower Society 1990].)

This is just a sample of the literature in bloodless medicine in the last few years.

In the field of medical ethics, progress has also been made. True, there still is ignorance on the subject of informed consent. A British editorialist noted

> the sad and troubling fact that many in society still do not know or understand the principles that comprise the law of consent for competent adults in England and Wales. . . . It is not for others to understand and approve or disapprove of the religious beliefs of anyone else; religion and faith is a personal feature of the lives of many, to the despair maybe of other members of the society who may not have a religious belief at all. . . . People have to recognize difference (alternative life beliefs and value systems) and be prepared if working as a health provider to concentrate on a professional and sensitive delivery of care that keeps personal opinions and beliefs where they have to remain—in the private domain of personal living. (Fullbrook 2007, p. 1306)

Using an interesting analogy in an article in the *Journal of Vascular Surgery*, the authors note that paternalistic instincts have "been trumped in the last century by common law and ethical theory that recognizes the surgeon as *an authority*, but places the patient *in authority* when decisions are made about his care. . . . A psychiatrist may not coerce or force an unwilling depressed patient requesting pharmacologic treatment to accept electroconvulsive therapy, even if the psychiatrist's long experience assures him that ECT will resolve the patient's condition more quickly and effectively" (Jones, McCullough, and Richman 2006, p. 422; italics in original).

A paper from Singapore concludes: "It is essential that the healthcare professionals respect the autonomy and decisions made by each Jehovah Witness patient, although it may not be in their best interests in the doctors' professional beliefs. . . . from the patient's perspective, it would seem to be in their best interests, with regard to respecting their spirituality and religious beliefs" (Chua and Tham 2006, p. 1000).

With this background, what is the best practical approach to the Jehovah's Witness patient? According to G. Effa-Heap, "good, honest communication, without any element of coercion or scare tactics" (2009, p. 176). Communication at the outset is important not only from the standpoint of maintaining good rapport. Equally critical is an initial understanding of the ground rules. An occasional source of frustration on the part of the clinician is the perception that each Witness "has a different position" on what is permissible. This has led to somewhat of a misconception that the Watchtower Society has changed or is changing the organizational policy on the matter of blood transfusion. In actuality, the society's direction has been essentially unchanged for decades. A position paper in the *Journal of the American Medical Association* in 1981 spelled out the basic stand that prevails today (Dixon and Smalley 1981).

Jehovah's Witnesses define a blood transfusion as one consisting of any of the main four components of blood, in addition to whole-blood transfusions. Are packed red cells a transfusion? Witnesses say yes. So are white cells, platelets, and plasma. But because blood can be fractionated in so many different ways, the decision beyond these four major components is left up to the individual conscience. The same position is taken regarding the proliferation of medical procedures and devices (cell-savers, heart-lung machines, etc.). Rather than making an organizational decree on each new thing that comes out, the decision is left to the conscience of the individual. Hence, the importance of open communication between clinician and patient from the start, so that the clinician can determine individual limits regarding blood fractions or medical procedures. Remark Sloan and Ballen, "Although these distinctions may seem artificial, caregivers should realize that most JWs are not merely submitting to an organizational mandate; they are earnestly striving to fulfill God's instructions" (Sloan and Ballen 2008).

To try to alleviate the confusion, the Witnesses have embarked on an internal educational campaign to keep their members as up to date as possible on their medical options and rights. Each Witness is encouraged to carry on his or her person a legal durable power of attorney or health care proxy listing health care agent, alternate, and end-of-life wishes. To the extent possible, this document delineates individual personal decisions on blood fractions and medical procedures.

In regard to the clinical strategies to follow with Jehovah's Witness patients, there are several fine recent reviews (Hughes, Ullery, and Barie 2008; Remmers and Speer 2006; Sniecinski and Levy 2007). All emphasize the importance of adequate preparation, a team approach, and comfortable experience with the many medical and surgical advances in bloodless techniques and medicines available. Wooley and Smith recommend a key strategy: "In otolaryngology, the best way to avoid the need for blood is to prevent acute haemorrhage. Careful tissue handling, recognition and avoidance of potential bleeding sources, and rapid control of haemorrhage are the best ways to achieve this aim. . . . If acute, severe haemorrhage does occur, the primary goal is to stop the bleeding" (Wooley and Smith 2007, p. 412). Though this seems so obvious, in the past many problems could have been avoided by aggressively combating delay in these patients.

Sometimes the delay may be in getting help. One U.S. paper recommends that "health care professionals seek assistance from others when they encounter conflicts with patients and families regarding treatment choices" (Brezina and Moskop 2007 p. 412). This is especially true when it comes to dealing with children of Witnesses. Though court orders can be obtained to administer blood transfusions over parents' objections in many parts of the world, there is increasing question whether this is always the best alternative, especially in light of more palatable options. There are now many bloodless pediatric centers willing to take babies and children as transfer patients, but this needs to be done in a timely fashion. A key resource is Hospital Information Services (his@wtbts.org, phone 718–560–4300), where an up-to-date medical consultant resource list is available 24 hours a day.

Another valuable source of assistance is the Hospital Liaison Committee, which the Witnesses have established locally for virtually all hospitals. The individuals who serve on these committees have been educated and trained to help alleviate confusion and apprehension that can arise in Witness medical situations. As mentioned in editorial correspondence regarding a difficult case in Britain, they "will not involve themselves in cases uninvited, but may, on request, assist in establishing the views and 'status' of patients presented as Witnesses" (Carter and Wade 2007, p. 90).

We can sum up where we started. In the words of Brezina and Moskop, "When professionals, patients, and parents express their opinions, beliefs, and guiding values, they can begin to seek common ground" (Brezina and Moskop 2007, p. 315).

Implications for the Practicing Physician

All medical practitioners who want to stay current will, over the course of a career, attend many postgraduate educational conferences. At these conferences, the latest medical evidence, advances, and recommendations will be presented. Though the contemporary clinical material will be presented as the "last word" on the subject, the astute clinician will soon recognize that what is meant really is the "latest word." And next year, or five years hence, the latest word may well be different.

This may seem obvious, but the implications for patient-doctor relationships can be staggering. In the 1980s and 90s, presentations to physicians on the value of estrogen supplementation for women were enthusiastic in outlining the myriad medical benefits and the extensive experimental backing. We enlightened physicians felt badly for our ignorant female patients who could not be convinced to avail themselves of this medical advance, these hormones. Then came the Women's Health Initiative study in 2002. Suddenly, our cautious, hesitant patients didn't seem so foolish anymore.

This example could be multiplied many times. For our discussion, let us consider the preponderant medical teaching on blood transfusions from the 1950s through the 1970s: the reassuring conferences on the safety of the nation's blood supply—until AIDS. Now we are repeatedly assured the blood supply is once again safe. We need to remember that is the latest word, not the last word.

We speak now to some general spiritual implications for the physician, not specific to the Jehovah's Witness patient.

The overriding point is that the practice of medicine is humbling. Each time the physician feels superiority when dealing with a patient who prefers "natural" treatment, or perhaps feels outrage with a patient who is for whatever reason not willing to follow scientific direction, that physician might well step back and treat himself or herself to a healthy dose of humility. In the end, in health matters, who really knows who is right?

Regarding medical wisdom, Osler expressed it poetically in "Aequanimitas": "In seeking absolute truth we aim at the unattainable, and must be content with finding broken portions. You remember in the Egyptian story . . . how they took the virgin Truth, hewed her lovely form into a thousand pieces, and scattered them to the four winds; . . . 'from that time ever since, the sad friends of truth . . . went up and down gathering up limb by limb still as they could find them. We have not yet found them all' " (Osler 1889, p. 7).

Years later, in the practice of medicine we still have not found them all, and we need to deal kindly with those who claim to have stumbled across a different piece from what we were looking for in our "double-blind studies." "To deal kindly"—indeed, this leads to the thrust of our discussion, How does spirituality enter into the doctor-patient relationship?

In Webster's *New World Dictionary*, the first definition for the word *spiritual* is "the spirit or the soul as distinguished from the body or material matters." As we have already seen, for Jehovah's Witnesses this definition is unacceptable because they feel the soul and the body are inextricably tied, there being no immortal something that leaves the body at death. But another definition of *spiritual* in Webster is "characterized by the ascendancy of the spirit; showing much refinement of thought and feeling." This is an interesting definition in the context of spirituality in the general doctor-patient relationship. This definition implies that the physician employs spirituality in the way he or she treats a patient. Appealing to Scripture, "The fruit of the Spirit is love, joy, peace, longsuffering, gentleness, goodness, faith, meekness, temperance" (Galatians 5:22–23, King James Bible). These simple qualities show how spirituality can enter the exam room when the physician opens the door.

Or again, consider the famous "Do for others what you want them to do for you" (Catholic Living Bible). The use of this Golden Rule helps define the spiritual physician. Isn't it what our patient asks for? Be kind to me. Show compassion. Be tolerant of my beliefs and foibles, for you may have one or two of your own.

Is there, then, a further way these spiritual qualities can be put to use to benefit our patient? Many think there is and that our profession is derelict in its duty. Francis W. Peabody said in 1927: "The most common criticism made at present by older practitioners is that young graduates have been taught a great deal about the mechanism of disease, but very little about the practice of medicine—or, to put it more bluntly, they are too 'scientific' and do not know how to take care of patients" (p. 877).

Now Peabody was a published and renowned scientist who believed a physician's first duty to a patient was the competent application of modern technology. And science is important in medicine. "Caring without science is well-intentioned kindness, but not medicine," says Bernard Lown (1996, cited in Rakel 2000, p. 442). To put it another way, "There is, thus, legitimate sense in the physician's claim that he knows better than his patient, what ails that patient" (Carson 1977, p. 1029). But after all the scientific lab tests, scans, and interventions have been performed, is there a further task for the physician? There is, and as we have defined *spiritual*, it is a spiritual task.

Back to Peabody. What if he could find nothing medically wrong with his patient, but the patient was still unwell? He spoke of a patient, Henry, who "is not disturbed so much by dyspnea as he is by anxiety for the future, and a talk with an understanding physician who tries to make the situation clear to him . . . does more to straighten him out than a book full of drugs and diets" (Peabody 1927, p. 879). His was a discussion of patients with what we would now call "functional complaints," and he estimated they constituted roughly half of the patients seeking medical attention in his day: "Medically speaking, they are not serious cases as regards prospective death, but they are often extremely serious as regards prospective life. Their symptoms will rarely prove fatal, but their lives will be long and miserable, and they may end by nearly exhausting their families and friends" (p. 879). A more contemporary physician, considering some patients who functioned well despite long-standing severe medical problems, noted: "You can be healed and still have a physically sick body. . . . And, I suppose, the reverse can be true. You can have no objectively demonstrable disease process and yet not be healthy and whole" (Mgebroff 2006, p. 42).

Here the role of the physician becomes spiritual, albeit to a limited degree. Says Peabody: "The successful diagnosis and treatment of these patients, however, depends almost wholly on the establishment of that intimate personal contact between physician and patient which forms the basis of private practice" (1927, p. 880). In the words of Anatole Broyard, "I wouldn't demand a lot of my doctor's time. I just wish he would brood on my situation for perhaps five minutes, that he would give me his whole mind just once, be bonded with me for a brief space, survey my soul as well as my flesh to get at my illness, for each man is ill in his own way" (Broyard 1994, cited in Rakel 2000, p. 444).

This then becomes the physician's second goal after professional medical ministrations. The physician has to be interested enough and empathetic enough to explain to the patient what is really wrong, even if it is not a physical problem, and make the patient believe it. This is the very province and privilege of the physician—to be admitted into the inner sanctum of the patient's being, to explore to the deepest secrets of the heart, and then to try, in some way, to help.

Does this not become a spiritual enterprise? Even further, returning now to our Jehovah's Witness patient who refuses a "life-saving" blood transfusion, we can now summarize spiritual principles that may on occasion affect other patients as well. Robert E. Rakel puts it this way: "Through empathy, physicians attempt to reconcile their own beliefs about what is best with the patient's beliefs. Without an empathetic approach, physicians risk harming patients by making decisions that are not congruent with their beliefs, values, and meaning of life as they perceive it. In addition, treating patients with tenderness and caring can relieve much of their emotional suffering and contribute more to their recovery than many of the drugs we use. . . . We must use the best technology that science has to offer, but never in a way that neglects the important emotional and social issues which make each patient unique" (Rakel 2000, p. 442).

In the words of Pope John Paul II, "violation of conscience is a grave act against man. It is the most painful blow inflicted on human dignity. It is, in a certain sense, worse than inflicting physical death, murder" (Pope John Paul II 1982).

Clearly, we as physicians share both the privilege and the responsibility to plumb some of the deepest spiritual issues that ever affect humans, our patients.

Conclusion

There may be one final spiritual nugget from our discussion of Jehovah's Witnesses. With all people, of whatever religion, in times of great stress as we often see in a medical setting, there is a universal constant that can be called on by anyone in extremis. It is this: the greatest force in the universe is—love. Just a few words, such as 1 Peter 5:7—"Throw all your anxiety upon him, because he cares for you" (New World Translation)—can be comforting, perhaps, to your dying patient.

You, doctor, will not change ultimately what will happen to your patient. The death rate in the world is still constant, 1:1. You can hope to change when it happens, but healing is related to wholeness. It's our job, not necessarily to cure, but to try to keep that person whole until death pays its call, whenever that may be.

The practice of medicine is humbling. The therapeutic miracles will be few and far between, and hard to come by. Oh, they will happen, and you will treasure each, but alas, they will be too infrequent to maintain your enthusiasm in the long run. The miracle will be not in the cure, but in the care. That may be the biggest lesson we as physicians can learn from Jehovah's Witnesses.

APPENDIX

Resources

Referrals, Consultations, Transfer of Care

Hospital Information Services: his@wtbts.org

24-hour emergency line: 718-560-4300 (up-to-date worldwide medical consultant resource list)

Jehovah's Witnesses Fact Sheet, 2008	
Worldwide Number of Baptized Witnesses	7,124,443
Number of Countries Reporting Witnesses	236
Number of Bloodless Medical Centers Worldwide	350
Worldwide Number of Hospital Liaison Committees	1,654

Sources: www.Watchtower.org; Hospital Information Services; Watchtower Society

REFERENCES

Adelola, O. A., I. Ahmed, and J. E. Fenton. 2008. Management of Jehovah's Witnesses in otolaryngology, head and neck surgery. *American Journal of Otolaryngology* 29:270–78.

Brezina, P. R., and J. C. Moskop. 2007. Urgent medical decision making regarding a Jehovah's Witness minor: A case report and discussion. *North Carolina Medical Journal* 68:312–16.

Broyard, A. 1994. *Intoxicated by My Illness*. New York: Random House.

Carson, R. A. 1977. What are physicians for? *JAMA* 238:1029–31.

Carter, R., and P. Wade. 2007. Jehovah's Witnesses: Who or what defines "best interests"? *Anesthesia* 62:90.

Casati, V., A. D'Angelo, L. Barbato, D. Turalla, F. Villa, M. A. Grasso, A. Porat, and F. Guerra. 2007. Perioperative management of four anaemic female Jehovah's Witnesses undergoing urgent complex cardiac surgery. *British Journal of Anaesthesia* 99:349–52.

Chua, R., and K. F. Tham. 2006. Will "no blood" kill Jehovah's Witnesses? *Singapore Medical Journal* 47:994–1002.

Digieri, L. A., I. P. Pistelli, and C. E. De Carvalho. 2006. The care of a child with multiple trauma and severe anemia who was a Jehovah's Witness. *Hematology* 11:187–191.

Dixon, J. L., and M. G. Smalley. 1981. Jehovah's Witnesses: The surgical/ethical challenge. *JAMA* 246:2471–72.

Effa-Heap, G. 2009. Blood transfusion: Implications of treating a Jehovah's Witness patient. *British Journal of Nursing* 18:174–77.

Fullbrook, S. 2007. Death by denomination: A Jehovah's right to die. *British Journal of Nursing* 16:1306–7.

Hughes, D. B., B. W. Ullery, and P. S. Barie. 2008. The contemporary approach to the care of Jehovah's Witnesses. *Trauma* 65:237–47.

Jeffrey, G. P., J. McCall, E. Gane, A. W. Mitchell, N. M. Gibbs, V. Beavis, K. Gunn, S. Munn, and A. K. House. 2007. Liver transplantation in Jehovah's Witness patients in Australasia. *Medical Journal of Australia* 187:188–89.

Jones, J. W., L. B. McCullough, and B. W. Richman. 2006. Painted into a corner: Unexpected complications in treating a Jehovah's Witness. *Journal of Vascular Surgery* 44:425–28.

Joseph, S. A. Jr., K. Berekashvili, M. M. Mariller, M. Rivlin, K. Sharma, A. Casden, F. Bitan, P. Kuflik, and M. Neuwirth. 2008. Blood conservation techniques in spinal deformity surgery: A retrospective review of patients refusing blood transfusion. *Spine* 33:2310–15.

King, C. E. 1982. *The Nazi State and the New Religions: Five Case Studies in Non-Conformity*. New York: Edwin Mellen Press.

Lown, B. 1996. *Lost Art of Healing*. New York: Houghton Mifflin.

Massiah, N., A. Athimulam, C. Loo, S. Okolo, and W. Yoong. 2007. Obstetric care of Jehovah's Witnesses: A 14-year observational study. *Archives of Gynecology and Obstetrics* 276:339–43.

Mgebroff, A. E. 2006. What my patients taught me about healing. *Medical Economics* 83:40–42.

Osler, W. 1889. Aequanimitas. Valedictory Address, University of Pennsylvania.

Pacsi, A. L. 2008. Case study: An ethical dilemma involving a dying patient. *Journal of the New York State Nurses Association* 39:4–7.

Peabody, F. W. 1927. The care of the patient. *JAMA* 88:877–82.

Pope John Paul II. 1982. Pope assails Polish loyalty oath. *St. Louis Post Dispatch,* 11 Jan., p. 12A.

Putney, L. J. 2007. Bloodless cardiac surgery: Not just possible, but preferable. *Critical Care Nursing Quarterly* 30:263–70.

Rakel, R. E. 2000. Compassion and the art of family medicine: From Osler to Oprah. *Journal of the American Board of Family Practice* 13:440–48.

Remmers, P. A., and A. J. Speer. 2006. Clinical strategies in the medical care of Jehovah's Witnesses. *American Journal of Medicine* 119:1013–18.

Sloan, J. M., and K. Ballen. 2008. SCT in Jehovah's Witnesses: The bloodless transplant. *Bone Marrow Transplantation* 41:837–44.

Sniecinski, R., and J. H. Levy. 2007. What is blood and what is not? Caring for the Jehovah's Witness patient undergoing cardiac surgery. *Anesthesia and Analgesia* 104:753–54.

Watchtower Society. 1990. *How Can Blood Save Your Life?* Watchtower Bible and Tract Society of Pennsylvania.

———. 2007. *What Does the Bible Really Teach?* Watchtower Bible and Tract Society of Pennsylvania.

———. 2008. *Yearbook of Jehovah's Witnesses*. Watchtower Bible and Tract Society of Pennsylvania.

———. 2009. Is all miraculous healing from God? *The Watchtower* 130:28.

Wooley, S. L., and D. R. K. Smith. 2006. ENT surgery, blood, and Jehovah's Witnesses. *Journal of Laryngology and Otology* 121:409–14.

CHAPTER ELEVEN

A Secular Perspective

David C. Ring, M.D., Ph.D.

For many of us, the scientific method (hypothesis formation, objective observation, and reproducible experiments) is the most constructive and fruitful way to address the human experience, particularly health and wellness. The spiritual aspects of illness can be considered equivalent to the psychological, sociological and behavioral aspects of medicine, all of which can be accounted for by using the scientific method. In this chapter I take the liberty of referring to spiritual aspects of health and illness in this way. The medical facts established by scientific experimentation are not typically disputed among various faiths and traditions. The realm of spirituality in medicine begins at the limits of science, at least when operating in the biomedical model of illness. The "art of medicine" may include both the necessary speculation at the limits of science as well as the differences between the biomedical and biopsychosocial aspects of illness. The spiritual aspects of medicine are what we do as individuals and communities at the limits of modern biomedical science to understand the difference between disease and illness—that is, between impairment (the objective pathophysiology) and disability (the impact on daily function and quality of life).

Insights about Life and Healing

Psychology

Psychology carries an undeserved stigma. Simply reading the word is likely to engender thoughts of flaws, weaknesses, and shame. We are often reluctant to admit that we are seeing a psychologist. We often fear or resent that a doctor might tell us that a physical complaint is "all in our heads."

Our society operates largely within a biomedical model of illness, according to which the solution to illness is finding and fixing the disease or pathophysiology. Because we are prone to all-or-none thinking, any discussion of the psychological aspects of illness seems to threaten our desired cure and we can quickly lose hope. For me, however, psychology greatly increases hope.

Psychology is the science of the human mind—how it works at its intelligent, rational, pattern-forming best. Of course, understanding the healthy workings of the mind can illuminate cognitive and behavioral processes that are dysfunctional as well, but the root of psychology, contrary to common conceptions, is positive.

When you stare at a two-dimensional drawing of a cube, your mind automatically tries to resolve the image into a three-dimensional object. As a result, your mind vacillates between seeing one or the other square as the front face of the cube. This action occurs at the level of neurons. It is hard-wired and cannot be changed. There is a basic ambiguity to our perceptions based on our anatomical structure.

If you look at a picture of two rectangles of the same size, with legs of a table drawn in with different orientations, your mind takes this additional information and interprets the rectangles as being of different sizes. This may be partly hard-wired and partly conditioned. In any case, the "extra information" contributes to the basic ambiguity of your perception.

As Tom Gilovich (1991) points out, humans tend to see patterns in everything, from the "hot hand" in basketball to bombing patterns in London during World War II. Our strength is to rationalize or make sense of things and see the patterns. This is what helps us to recognize faces better than a computer can, but it is also what makes us easy targets for charlatans. An easy, passive, external path to wellness holds great appeal, and we are tempted by anything that offers a convincing rationale.

Investment in belief and meaning is a powerful healer, as seen in the placebo effect. This, as well as the tendency of things to regress to the mean and the self-limiting course of many symptoms and diseases, are reasons why a treatment may "work" aside from any direct effect on pathophysiology. This has been most clearly demonstrated in clinical trials involving sham surgery, such as the trial that compared sham surgery, simple washout, and debridement during arthroscopic treatment of knee arthritis and found no differences in outcome between the three groups.

An appreciation for the workings of the human mind improves our understanding of the differences between disease and illness and between impairment and disability (Vranceanu, Barsky, and Ring 2009). Illness and illness behavior are complex products of biological, psychological, sociological, and behavioral factors. Each of the various aspects of illness presents opportunities for increasing health and wellness. An understanding of the human mind opens up these possibilities for doctors and their patients.

In some ways, a focus on science rather than on faith and tradition may facilitate consideration of these "spiritual" aspects of illness. Just as somatoform disorders arise in part because it is more acceptable to have a physical complaint than to admit depression, anxiety, or stress (Barsky and Borus 1999), faith and faith traditions can provide a convenient means for sidestepping the need to accept and adapt to the inherent uncertainty and limitations of knowledge, including medical knowledge. Just as the scientist comes to feel exhilarated rather than threatened by the need for experimentation to overcome the shortcomings of his or her intelligent mind, we can all become comfortable with puzzlement, uncertainty, and limitations without losing hope and while still having a fulfilling and enjoyable life. In other words, science and the scientific method provide comfort and hope, which some might argue are the most sought-after benefits of faith. In this way, some of us find no role for faith or religion in our spiritual lives.

Intuition

Intuition, automatic thoughts, "gut feelings"—we all appreciate the degree to which these serve us well. Some of us do not appreciate how much trouble they can get us into. From a scientific perspective, intuition is a product of biology or genetics, experience, and training (Gladwell 2005). When there is little time for experimentation, our gut feelings can help us make the correct judgment and the correct decision. Physicians use intuition (heuristics) deftly to make decisions where there is neither time nor complete data for a more measured consideration, but intuition can also cause physicians to overlook less common or unexpected diagnoses, to the detriment of the patient (Groopman 2007).

Thus, intuition can be a great help or a great hindrance. The mind's pattern-forming and rationalizing instincts are both its greatest power and its most important weakness (Gladwell 2005; Groopman 2007). Magicians use these instincts to fool us—they know how to use our minds' pattern-forming instincts to distract (Randi 1982). Our attention is in one place while the trick is performed somewhere else. Magicians prefer an intelligent audience, because well-functioning minds are easier to fool with sleight of hand. It is against the magician's ethic to claim supernatural powers; theirs is the art of deception—deception of the intelligent, highly functioning human mind. Intuition should be respected for its role in allowing us to deftly navigate the real world, but it should not be followed blindly.

Perhaps most important, intuition can be trained. Just as getting fit requires an investment in dieting and exercise, cultivating a more adaptive, resilient, and positive intuition takes effort and dedication (Gladwell 2002). The expertise provided by those who best understand the mind—mental health professionals, and specifically cognitive behavioral therapists—can be invaluable (Vranceanu, Barsky, and Ring 2009).

The Scientific Tradition

Science is what humans use to put their intuition to the test, to avoid fooling themselves or being fooled by others (Sagan 1996). It acknowledges the basic ambiguity of human perception, our strong pattern-forming instincts, and the influence of ego and authority.

Just as "chance favors the prepared mind," the willingness to question one's intuition is a key to good health. Many if not most medical advancements have been through "happy accidents" (Myers 2007). They were counterintuitive and benefited from researchers' having open minds and a willingness to question gut feelings, faith, and traditions.

While those in poor countries still suffer disproportionately from diseases that can be addressed with sanitation, public safety, effective medications, and surgery, most of us in the resource-rich world die of diseases of senescence such as cancer and heart disease. A substantial proportion of disability in the resource-rich parts of the world correlates with misconceptions about symptoms or illnesses, many of which are colored by depression, most of them reinforced by unrealistic expectations coming from media and popular culture. Science measures this; it explains this; and it can help determine the best methods for ameliorating it (Vranceanu, Barsky, and Ring 2009).

From the secular point of view, faith is employed at the limits of modern science. Faith—believing that one knows or understands something in the absence of sufficient experimental evidence—is often counterproductive. Faith in the sense of optimal "spiritual" health, on the other hand, is an integral part of wellness in a way that is measurable by experiment.

Relationship to Contemporary Medical Practice

A social construct exists because the members of a society agree to behave as if it exists, according to Wikipedia. Examples of social constructs include constructs of gender, value, beauty, and social stature such as the caste system in India. In medicine, consumption is an example of an illness construct that was used to explain the syndrome produced by tuberculosis. An integral part of this illness construct was a speculative etiology, most commonly the foul city air. Once Koch's elegant scientific experimentation demonstrated that consumption reflected the pathophysiology associated with infection by *Mycobacterium tuberculosis*, the illness construct of consumption disappeared: it was no longer needed (King 1952).

Some of the most common illnesses have no identifiable pathophysiology and exist only as syndromes and illness constructs (Vranceanu, Barsky, and Ring 2009; Masi 1998). The pathophysiology of some of these will one day be explained, but many are likely prove to be somatoform disorders—an overinterpretation and overreaction to symptoms that are not associated with underlying pathophysiology (Vranceanu, Barsky, and Ring 2009; Gladwell 2005). Historical examples include the illness known as hysteria (now known as conversion disorder), which paralyzed innumerable young women in the latter part of the nineteenth century. After Babinski and others developed objective tests for upper motor neuron pathology, this culturally conditioned disorder largely disappeared (Shorter 1992).

The scientist is comfortable with the fact that we cannot currently verify or falsify some of our most common illnesses. We are open to the possibility that diseases such as fibromyalgia, chronic fatigue syndrome, and multiple chemical sensitivity, among others, may turn out to be verifiable diseases (pathophysiological processes) or may be full-fledged somatoform disorders or something in between. Those who are more confident about one of the formulations of these illness concepts are basing that confidence on faith alone—specifically, on an overvaluing of their intuition.

Charlatanism has always been rampant. Much is for personal profit, while some purveyors actually have faith in their wares. Arguably, charlatans in the latter category do more harm (Randi 1982). The scientist does not believe in any treatment or intervention. Either experiments can demonstrate that a treatment is better than placebo, regression to the mean, or the self-limiting course of the illness, or they cannot. If the usefulness of a treatment cannot be demonstrated by experiment, if it cannot be verified or falsified, than it is unlikely to be worth the expenditure of resources and hope.

In the absence of viable alternatives it is reasonable to place some faith and hope in unproved treatments, but one should always be honest with oneself and with others about this process. To knowingly use the placebo effect by claiming greater confidence or certainty than is warranted is deceptive and unethical (Ernst and Singh 2008). In essence, one should be honest about the fact that we are using creative speculation and imagination to bolster our spiritual health: we are using our confidence, optimism, self-efficacy, and well-being. The scientist seeks the benefits of the placebo effect without the deception. Evidence suggests that training our intuition using techniques such as cognitive behavioral therapy can achieve this (Vranceanu, Barsky, and Ring 2009).

How Beliefs Influence Practice

From the secular point of view, the spirituality of medicine lies in the difference between disease (objectively verifiable pathophysiology) and illness (the individual's experience of the disease). In the traditional biomedical model of medicine, there is little distinction between disease and illness. Thus, if one has painful trapeziometacarpal arthrosis (arthritis at the base of the thumb), the symptoms will correlate with the severity of the disease; and medication, splints, or surgery to address the arthritis are the only ways to improve health and wellness. In contrast, the biopsychosocial behavioral model of medicine acknowledges that among the millions of people with trapeziometacarpal arthrosis (it's a normal and inevitable part of aging), a small percentage present to the doctor with complaints, and a small percentage of those patients request surgery. The same disease creates a disabling illness in some and a minor nuisance consistent with a rich and healthy life in others, with most of us falling somewhere in between (Vranceanu, Barsky, and Ring 2009).

Consider the distinction between nociception and pain. Nociception is the physiology of pain. The chemicals and nerve signals presented to the brain or mind. Pain is what the individual does with those nociceptive signals. The massive divide between pain and nociception is evident in the stories of battlefield or athletic heroism.

The differences between impairment (objectively measurable dysfunction) and disability (what a person perceives him- or herself as incapable of doing) are also heartening. We are all touched by the stories of people who have amputations or other severe injuries or illness achieving at a high level, and as an orthopedic surgeon I have the privilege of witnessing these heroes every day. On the other hand, a large proportion of our society is disproportionately disabled in spite of little or no objectively verifiable pathology (Vranceanu, Barsky, and Ring 2009; Groopman 2004). I try to limit medical and surgical interventions to those conditions that have a strong evidence base. In all settings I emphasize the importance of peace of mind, a sense of wellness, self-efficacy, and resiliency.

The divide between disability and impairment has been consistently explained in large part by depression, misconceptions about or over-interpretation of symptoms, and health anxiety or heightened illness concern (the state of being convinced that you are seriously ill). It has been noted that at a time when our objective situation is better than ever, our overall happiness is actually decreasing—a phenomenon that Easterbrook (2004) refers to as the progress paradox.

Addressing and Accessing Spirituality in Practice

Before you begin to lose hope, science comes to the rescue. There is extensive experimental evidence that cognitive behavioral therapies (learning to understand your intuition or automatic thoughts, to see the value of questioning them, and then to train an optimally adaptive and resilient intuition) can improve health and wellness (Vranceanu, Barsky, and Ring 2009). A thorough understanding and appreciation of these aspects of health and wellness should convince us to insist on the most positive, optimistic, enabling, practical, resourceful illness concepts and constructs consistent with the best available evidence. We should resist any negative illness concepts until the experimental evidence is strong—I would argue that we should resist until the evidence is irrefutable (Myers 2007; Lozano-Calderon, Anthony, and Ring 2008).

In my practice, I connect with patients by active listening, empathy, and legitimization of their concerns. If a safe and caring relationship is established, I try to help them consider the opportunities offered by the biopsychosocial model of medicine. The first step is seeing the value of questioning one's automatic thoughts and intuition.

The Relationship between a Secular Perspective and Culture

The scientific culture is comfortable with uncertainty and places emphasis on the ability to make predictions about manipulation of the environment based on consistent confirmation of hypotheses. Scientists love to be proved wrong—indeed, to prove their own theories incorrect—because ultimately they seek the reproducible objective facts that allow us to understand and manipulate our environment. The success of this approach leads one to feel that life and health are optimized in the absence of faith. Science alone establishes the importance of spiritual health.

REFERENCES

Barsky, A. J., and J. F. Borus. 1999. Functional somatic syndromes. *Annals of Internal Medicine* 130:910 21.

Easterbrook, G. 2004. *The Progress Paradox: How Life Gets Better While People Feel Worse*. New York: Random House.

Ernst, E., and S. Singh. 2008. *Trick or Treatment: The Undeniable Facts about Alternative Medicine*. New York: W.W. Norton.

Gilovich, T. 1991. *How We Know What Isn't So: The Fallibility of Human Reason in Everyday Life*. New York: Free Press.

Gladwell, M. 2005. *Blink: The Power of Thinking without Thinking*. New York: Little, Brown.

Groopman, J. 2007. *How Doctors Think*. New York: First Mariner.

King, L. S. 1952. Dr. Koch's postulates. *Journal of the History of Medicine and Allied Sciences* 7:350–61.

Lozano-Calderón, S., S. Anthony, and D. Ring. 2008. The quality and strength of evidence for etiology: Example of carpal tunnel syndrome. *Journal of Hand Surgery—American* 33:525–38.

Masi, A. T. 1998. Concepts of illness in populations as applied to fibromyalgia syndromes: A biopsychosocial perspective. *Zeitschrift für Rheumatologie* 57, Suppl. 2: 31–35.

Myers, M. 2007. *Happy Accidents: Serendipity in Modern Medical Breakthroughs*. New York: Arcade Publishing.

Randi, J. 1982. *Flim-Flam! Psychics, ESP, Unicorns, and Other Delusions*. New York: Prometheus.

Sagan, C. 1996. *The Demon-Haunted World: Science as a Candle in the Dark*. New York: Random House.

Shorter, E. 1992. *From Paralysis to Fatigue: A History of Psychosomatic Illness in the Modern Era*. New York: Free Press.

Vranceanu, A. M., A. Barsky, and D. Ring. 2009. Psychosocial aspects of disabling musculoskeletal pain. *Journal of Bone and Joint Surgery—American* 91:2014–18.

PART III / Implications and Applications

CHAPTER TWELVE

Ethical Considerations and Implications for Professionalism

Michael J. Balboni, M.Div., Th.M., Ph.D.; Terry R. Bard, D.D.; Shan W. Liu, M.D., S.D.; Michael N. D'Ambra, M.D.; Travis D. Johnson, M.D., M.P.H.; Walter Moczynski, D.Min., M.T.S., M.Div.; and John R. Peteet, M.D.

> The most important problem for the future of professionalism is neither economic nor structural but cultural and ideological. The most important problem is its soul. ELIOT FREIDSON (2001, P. 213)

We have seen in preceding chapters how spirituality can shape the values of physicians, and how they understand their role. In this chapter we consider the implications of differing spiritual and secular perspectives for several questions that are often contested: the basis of professionalism, the relationship between a physician's personal and professional identity, the boundaries of a physician's role, the conscientious refusal of care, and the therapeutic use of spiritual interventions. The contrasting positions pro and con that follow demonstrate the complexity of the issues at stake.

Pro 1: Professionalism Is Spiritually Based

There is always a tension between the needs of the physician and the needs of the patient, as Jonsen outlines below:

> A profound moral paradox pervades medicine. That paradox arises from the incessant conflict of the two most basic principles of morality: self-interest and altruism. Certainly, every human being feels, from time to time, the tug of these principles. Every profession and occupation is marked, to some extent, by the

> tension. But the opposition is, I believe, built into the very structure of medical care and woven into the fabric of physicians' lives. The many particular moral problems encountered in medicine are symptoms of this profound paradox. Many of the social and economic features of medical care are, in some way, outgrowths of this paradox. Many of the psychological troubles of physicians (and their families) are fomented by the inability to manage the pressures of this paradox. Of course, I cannot support these assertions with solid epidemiologic studies or statistically impressive empirical research. I merely propose them as the reflections of a sympathetic and experienced doctor watcher. (Jonsen 1983, p. 1532)

Society has traditionally deferred regulation of this tension to the medical profession, assuming that it honors this deference by self-regulation of its members. However, the past decade has seen a resurgence in the development and teaching of professionalism, due to a perceived decline in professionalism. This decline has several causes: As medicine has become more dependent on technology, physicians spend less time relating to their patients. Commercialism has increased the conflicts between the interests of patients and physicians. The intrusion of third parties such as managed care organizations into the physician-patient relationship have heightened this conflict (Huddle 2005). In Coulehan's words, the result has been that "while the minds of our students became sharper than ever, their hearts appeared listless, and their moral compasses adrift" (2005, p. 893). In response, many professional organizations have drafted statements on professionalism (American Board of Internal Medicine 2002). Medical educators have also tried to instill more professionalism through traditional didactics and evaluating students and residents as they progress through their training.

There are multiple reasons why this approach is likely to be insufficient. One is that it is not a knowledge deficit that leads to lack of professionalism, but the difficulty of continually juggling the array of demands that physicians experience. Most physicians know that they should empathize more, listen more, or explain more to their patients. However, with today's busy schedules, providing the ideal competent, compassionate care comes at the cost of adequate rest, bathroom breaks, eating lunch, or even seeing all of the other patients in a timely fashion. Additionally, there are strong narratives within the hospital culture that teach an "informal curriculum," which undermine optimal care (Coulehan 2005). Perhaps most importantly, the movement fails to address the role that spirituality plays in the formation of a professional.

Huddle contends that "in asking for professionalism, that is, for just, altruistic, conscientious and compassionate physicians and trainees, medical educators are asking for morality, which is at bottom asking for more than expertise" (2005, p. 886). The core of professionalism is rooted not only in "what shall I do" but "who am I" as a physician. If indeed, how to increase professionalism in medicine is less about teaching ethical reasoning in complex cases, and more about how to encourage physicians to continue to navigate through their careers with a continued spirit of altruism and compassion, we then postulate that a discussion of professionalism is remiss unless it includes spirituality.

Spirituality holds an important place in (1) the historical and central root of what it means to be professional, (2) the intimately intertwined role that religion and spirituality have in oaths, and (3) the resources important to physicians in their professional journeys. Essentially, the field of medicine may increase professionalism by creating professionals whose development is intimately involved with their own spirituality. While spirituality is not the only basis of professionalism, it can be an important one to many physicians. Spirituality is better nurtured by mentoring and by involvement in spiritual communities than by didactic teaching; beyond that, each professional should take responsibility for the deepening of his or her own spirituality.

The Roots of Professionalism

The Merriam-Webster dictionary defines *professionalism* as "the conduct, aims or qualities that . . . mark a profession or a professional person." The word *profession*, in turn, can refer to

1. the act of taking the vows of a religious community;
2. an act of openly declaring or publicly claiming a belief, faith, or opinion: protestation;
3. an avowed religious faith;
4. a. a calling requiring specialized knowledge and often long and intensive academic preparation;
   b. a principal calling, vocation, or employment;
   c. the whole body of persons engaged in a calling.

According to Ronald Labonte, a professor of globalization and health equity, "The Latin root of the word *professional* means to 'profess' or 'vow,' a reference to the medieval practice of surrendering personal gain to the larger community of a religious order or worker's guild" (Minkler 2005, p. 86).

Historically, then, the root of the word *professionalism* has links to religion and faith. Likewise, it involves subjugating one's personal interest to the interest of the patient and to the community of one's peers in medicine. Like other professions, medicine has traditionally been based in spiritual and community roots. Therefore, for historical reasons, it is important to address the spiritual roots of professionalism. We do not claim that modern-day professionalism has to address spirituality simply for historical reasons. Instead, we postulate that there are valid reasons why professionalism has been rooted in spirituality that remain relevant.

Oaths in Medicine

An oath is "a performative utterance with moral weight that encumbers the speaker" and has five essential qualities (Sulmasy 1999b, p. 331). First, it calls on a higher power to assist the professors of the oath to perform their duties listed within the oath. Second, it binds the professor to another individual or group in a significant, if not spiritual, way. Third, it recognizes that this binding is a higher calling from the higher power and is above the capability of the individual. Fourth, the oath recognizes that such a binding before the higher power causes a transformation in the essence of the individual that enables him or her to fulfill the calling. Last, the oath calls on the professor to be accountable to the higher power and to the witnesses of the oath to carry out the vow.

Oaths in medicine, which have been used throughout history to define and defend the aims of the profession, follow the outline given by Sulmasy (1999b) and reflect an intimate connection between professionalism and spirituality. The original oath describing the ethics of medicine is attributed to Hippocrates circa 460 BCE (Medical Oaths 2009). Other cultures have followed suit with oaths that represent their own cultural and religious values. Significant historical oaths from different cultures and times include the Prayer and Oath of Maimonides, written in the 13th century; Thomas Sydenham's challenge to physicians in 1668; and the Oath of a Muslim Physician, compiled in 1976 (Hippocratic Registry 2008). Examining traditional oaths reveals that the forebearers of medicine sought spiritual guidance to enable physicians to professionally care for their patients.

Interestingly, these oaths anticipated struggles similar to those that have brought about the resurgence in teaching professionalism today. They recognize that medicine is a high calling that binds patients and physicians in a special healing relationship. This relationship may be conflicted by the potential for personal sacrifice on the part of the physician and by great temptation for self-gain. To safeguard such a relationship, the oaths appeal to spiritual deities to uplift the character of physicians to enable them to fulfill their professional responsibilities.

The oaths define the relationship between the physician and the patient as a spiritual calling, requiring a commitment of their very lives. The Jewish scholar Maimonides states that it is the duty of the physician to care for God's creation. Thomas Sydenham, known as "the English Hippocrates," declared that God has entrusted patients' lives to the physicians, thus requiring that they give themselves with all diligence to the care of patients. The oath of the Muslim physician calls for physicians to devote their lives to their patients. As a result, the physician's life is different and is no longer his or her own.

The goal of an oath is the transformation of the person to enable the person to fulfill his or her calling. It is a commitment to change one's integrity, values, and aims in the light of current circumstances. Traditionally, the depth of change an oath requires necessitates the help of a power greater than the speaker or the public to whom the person is speaking (Sulmasy 1999b). Being entrusted with the care of another person's life is an overwhelming responsibility. In addition, the temptation is great to take advantage of medical knowledge for personal gain. These two burdens compel the oath taker to call on a greater power for support. Hippocrates calls on Apollo and the pantheon of all gods and goddesses for help. The oath of a Muslim physician asks Allah for wisdom to treat patients and strength to refrain from the temptation of the abomination of idolatry. Maimonides recognizes that eternal providence appointed the physician, and his oath requests that avarice, miserliness, and glory not engage the physician's mind. Sydenham's first directive is that the doctor must give account to the Supreme Judge for all his care. He also calls for all actions of the doctor to be for God's glory and not his or her own.

It is apparent that each of these oaths sees the first step toward professionalism as the recognition that the physician is not the ultimate authority in life and therefore needs the help of a greater power to perform his or her calling. Maimonides finishes his oath by stating, "Here am I ready for my vocation and now I turn to my calling." There is an almost a palpable burden taken on in this statement. In taking their oath, physicians vow before God to care for his creatures at the expense of their own ambitions. Knowing this cost, they turn from their old ways and walk forward with a new profession. They have been changed. Acknowledging such a burdensome request, the oath of Muslims requests that Allah change them to be worthy of such a calling.

These oaths make clear that the profession of medicine requires a binding to a vocation that changes the life, ambitions, and direction of the physician once he has turned to follow this calling. Each of these oaths declares to the public the values of medicine, proclaims to the young doctor the expectations of the profession, and commits him or her to maintain the deep heritage that defines medicine (Smith 1996), a heritage of using knowledge and skills to benefit patients and the community (Coller, Klotman, and Smith 2002). Ultimately, a medical oath establishes "an expectation of altruism, of effacement of self-interest" and "of trustworthy fidelity." "As a performative utterance," Sulmasy continues, " it makes the doctor of medicine a physician" (Sulmasy 1999b, p. 341).

The critical role of spirituality in guiding medical practice is codified in the American Medical Association's first code of medical ethics, which states, "Medical Ethics as a branch of General Ethics must rest on the basis of religion and morality."

Spirituality as a Resource for Physicians

In addition to helping to define a physician's calling, spirituality is a resource for physicians in achieving professionalism and in dealing with the stresses of professional life. One all-too-common example of such stress is being the subject of a medical malpractice lawsuit. The complaint is served by a sheriff, and from the very start, one is made to feel like a criminal. Physicians are often emotionally devastated when this happens, fearing that they will be reported to the state board and the national registry, and as a result will lose their retirement savings, their home, and their ability to move their practice to another hospital or state. Many hospitals provide stress management resources such as counseling and groups to support physicians going through the process. The lawyers assigned to the case usually offer to be available to answer questions and address concerns, but at the same time they tell physicians that this process will take 3 to 5 years to resolve. For many physicians, the guilt, the shame, the uncertainty, and the total lack of control is disruptive to their day-to-day practice and to their personal well-being (Charles, Wilbert, and Franke 1985). For those physicians with spiritual faith that an outside power is capable of answering prayer, the relief of stress and worry can be profound. If the physician is capable of "handing over the fear and worry" to this outside power, the burden is lifted, and it becomes easier to go forward with life and work during the long period of waiting.

Spirituality as a Source of Values

Kinghorn and colleagues (2007) point out that students who enter medical training fluent in the moral aspects of professionalism do so because they have learned in "familial, cultural and/or religious communities, often from an early age, to value the virtues of respect, altruism, and service." Rather than ignoring these sources of morality, those seeking to foster professionalism should encourage students and trainees to reflect on where they can find support for their moral values as they progress through their medical careers. If these moral values are not nurtured, students and physicians run the risk of losing integrity and of experiencing conflict between their personal and professional identities.

Spirituality as a Source of Strength for Being Professional

Beyond being an important source of values for physicians, spiritual communities can provide continued support for living them out, counterbalancing the influences of medical culture that may cause students to regress in moral development (Lind 2000) or cause house staff to burn out (Shanafelt et al. 2002) or become cynical (Griffith and Wilson 2003). Larkin, McKay, and Angelos (2005) address an inherent tension and challenge to professionalism: self-care and moral nurturing throughout the professional life cycle are particularly important in times of ballooning public expectation, malpractice crises, increased time pressures, workforce shortages, decreased reimbursement, and increasingly managed care. Overworked doctors do "bad" things not because they are inherently bad or do not know scientific principles or lack common sense, but because they are tired or exhausted and are so busy performing an endless cycle of documentation that they miss out on talking fully with their patients.

Those who enter the field of medicine are generally idealistic and desire to care for others. However, the increasing demands of the job make it more and more difficult always to act professionally. It is here— when physicians are fatigued but still need to be patient, when they are confronted with belligerent patients but still need to treat everyone with dignity, when they are tempted to take an easier but morally questionable route—that faith and spirituality may help them cope and thus be a source of strength. Because the behavior of physicians is largely self-regulated, encouraging them to seek as many resources as possible, including spiritual ones, will, one hopes, increase their ability not only to continue to strive to be professional, but also to find more lifelong career satisfaction.

Spirituality as a Resource for Moral Failure

Spiritual traditions provide ways of finding forgiveness. Because physicians' expectations of themselves are often unrealistic, they can be pushed to the point of burnout when they make mistakes, or can fail to act professionally. In especially challenging situations, such as when they are being sued, physicians are more likely to be depressed and angry and feel defeated (Charles, Wilbert, and Franke 1985). Confession, sharing one's failures with others in a community supportive of one's values, and asking for forgiveness can be helpful antidotes. Spirituality also facilitates discovering purpose in a physician's life. Spiritual transformation allows healing, growth, and freedom from the obligation to function as a god.

Spirituality and Public Health

On a broader level, spirituality can also play a large role in motivating physicians to think even beyond the benefit of the individual patient, to consider improving the public health. There is concern that certain groups may and do use the provision of health care as a means to proselytize. In such cases the individual's or the organization's motives beyond the provision of medical care may present an ethical dilemma.

We have outlined how the inherent tension between altruism and self-interest has created a need for the medical field to create declarations of professionalism and have suggested that current strategies for fostering professionalism, while laudable, are likely to be ineffective. Including spirituality in the discussion may help not only because of its historical importance in defining what it means to be a professional, but also because of the resource it provides physicians in becoming professional persons. To other suggested means of fostering professionalism, such as encouraging mentorship, changing hospital narratives, requiring community service, and engaging in moral communities (Coulehan 2005; Huddle 2005; Kinghorn et al. 2007; Larkin, McKay, and Angelos 2005), we would add deepening the physician's spiritual journey.

Con 1: Professionalism Is Not Spiritually Based

A number of books by atheists such as Dawkins (2006), Hitchens (2007), and Stenger (2008) point out the irrationality and immorality of much that is done in the name of religion. Scientists such as Dawkins further emphasize the danger of acting on the belief that one is representing God and the need to subject all human ideas to objective scrutiny. Physicians who link their sense of professionalism to divine inspiration need to exercise caution about the possibility that they could be listening to their own projected wishes or ideals. As David Ring suggests earlier in this volume, the honesty and integrity valued by secularists is central to the practice of good medicine because so many patients want to believe in unproven, potentially harmful promises of cure.

While religious believers have long claimed that morality is comprehensible and sustainable only in relation to a transcendent source (God), evolutionary explanations for morality are now widely accepted (Sinnott-Armstrong 2009). At the level of the individual, important sources of morality other than religious faith include the concepts that one learns from one's family upbringing, reading, and colleagues. Sociologists such as Phil Zuckerman (2008) point out that secular societies such those in Denmark, France, Hong Kong, Japan, Norway, and Sweden are among the most affluent, egalitarian, peaceful, and happy. These countries, which rely on the belief that people can be good without God, seem not to need God to care effectively for the health of their citizens.

Finally, making faith an explicit part of the medical workplace (for example, in oaths expected of all) can easily discriminate, making atheists or agnostics uncomfortable. A better basis for shared professional ethics can be found in the Dalai Lama's response to a question about the sources of his inspiration. He described "human values" that unite us: "I call these secular ethics, secular beliefs. There's no relationship with any particular religion. Even without religion, even as nonbelievers, we have the capacity to promote these things" (Pal 2006).

Pro 2: Physicians Should Keep Private Their Personal Spiritual or Religious Identities

A physician should generally avoid making personal statements, religious or otherwise, in the clinical setting, for at least three reasons. First, the physician's responsibility is to serve the needs of the patient, not his own or some other agenda. Apart from the ethical risk of actual proselytizing, the differential of power that exists between patient and physician makes the potential for undue influence in communicating his beliefs and affiliations inescapable. Second, even wearing a religious symbol such as a cross or a yarmulke can present a distraction, if not an offense. Some patients may feel unable to accept care from a physician whom they see as representing a group that has oppressed them or their family. Third, spiritual commitments that are allowed to intrude into the physician's work life can present problems for fellow trainees and colleagues, who must bear the burden of increased weekend or holiday call. Some Orthodox Jews have appropriately selected specialties such as radiology that allow them to minimize these burdens on others.

Con 2: Physicians Should Share Their Personal Spiritual or Religious Identities

There are clearly risks to personal disclosure of any kind in the clinical encounter, and physicians need to make decisions about disclosure guided by what serves the patient. At the same time, patients often want a physician to recommend a course of action as a person, as well as an expert in disease. Patients who ask for a physician's advice need informed consent about the physician's values. On morally controversial issues such as abortion, homosexuality, or assisted suicide, they especially need and deserve transparency about the worldview or spirituality that informs the physician's response to their questions. A physician whose person or office indicates a religious identification is being proactively transparent and open to questions, which is ethically very different from imposing or proselytizing.

One useful way to think about the impact of dual loyalties on professional boundaries is to distinguish between "boundary crossing," a descriptive term, and "boundary violation," which is a harmful crossing or transgression of a boundary. As Gutheil and Gabbard (1993) note, the specific impact of a boundary crossing can be assessed only by careful attention to the clinical context. For example, it could be coercive and unethical to suggest prayer to a patient, but depending on the clinical context, it could be therapeutic to accept a patient's request to pray together if a clinician could do so sincerely and with a clear understanding of how it advances the goals of the treatment.

The power differential in the therapeutic relationship makes attention to boundaries necessary, but clinicians can work to reduce this power differential by encouraging more mutual relationships in treatment (Blackshaw and Miller 1994). The Massachusetts Board of Registration in Medicine's 1994 guidelines for boundaries in psychotherapy point out that while self-disclosure should generally be kept to a minimum in psychotherapy, there are occasions in which self-disclosure is appropriate (e.g., discussion of the physician's training and qualifications), and infrequent occasions when self-disclosure can have an important therapeutic impact. The guidelines note: "These situations need to be well thought out, and it must be clear that these disclosures serve the patient, not the therapist" (Massachusetts Board 1994, p. 5).

A physician who has been asked to see a member of his or her same congregation as a patient should consider the potential impact on their relationship imposed by their kinship in the faith, and its meaning: Is this the only way that a patient will trust a physician? Is the patient seeking to establish a special connection with the clinician that will make therapeutic objectivity more difficult to maintain? If the patient is being referred by a respected figure in his church hierarchy, will the physician feel pressure to treat the patient differently? Anticipating, discussing, and maintaining confidentiality become particularly important in such situations.

Finally, physicians need to consider whether informed consent exists for working in this sensitive area of their patients' lives. For example, to decide whether they can trust a physician with information about issues such as abortion, homosexuality, or moral failure, patients may want to know whether the physician shares their basic values and orientations to life. Some patients may want to know more than physicians feel comfortable in sharing. One potentially helpful question in knowing how to proceed is: "If I explore further your spiritual concerns (or tell you my own religious identification, or join you in a prayer, or suggest a church for you to try) how will it help with our work of getting you better?" Without clarity on this basic question— the therapeutic rationale for boundary crossing—it will be difficult to establish informed consent.

Pro 3: Provision of Spiritual Care Is within the Boundaries of the Physician's Role

While no one disagrees that physicians should focus on the material aspects of illness, respect patients' wishes, and provide excellent technical care, a strong argument can be made that their competence should also extend to understanding the patient as a person, including his or her spiritual and religious dimensions. Illness raises profound challenges within every sphere of human experience including the spiritual, mental, social, and physical (Sulmasy 2002). These dimensions of personhood intersect with one another and cannot be easily separated. Health services need to provide seamless care that addresses all aspects of a patient's illness.

Proponents of spiritual inquiry encourage physicians to identify needs and refer patients to religious and spiritual professionals (Lo et al. 2002; Scheurich 2003; Puchalski 2008). While there are benefits in efficiency and expertise brought by a division of labor in a complex economic and social health system, strict adherence to a disciplinary division of labor fails to take into account the ways in which the biomedical and the spiritual overlap and influence one another. Consider the case of a 44-year-old, highly committed Roman Catholic man who has terminal cancer and is contemplating aggressive treatment. He rejects his physician's counsel to transition to palliative care. He seriously considers experimental treatments and alternative therapies because he believes that God has given him the responsibility to care for his two adolescent daughters until they reach adulthood.

When the material and spiritual directly intersect in this way, physicians and nurses are uniquely positioned to address and possibly provide appropriate spiritual support (Balboni and Balboni 2010; Balboni et al. 2010). Circumscribed boundaries (e.g., leaving such concerns to a chaplain) intended to protect patient autonomy may limit the degree of spiritual support available to such patients and worsen medical outcomes. All this suggests two significant changes that could move religion and spirituality away from the margins of health care. First, pastoral care and chaplaincy services should be further expanded and integrated into the health care team as modeled in palliative care. Multidisciplinary care of patients allows for distinct disciplines to realize a more robust practice of care and cure for the whole patient. It also encourages individual team members to think in an interdisciplinary way. Second, spiritual care must also be democratized in a medical context. Spiritual care should not be conceived as purely a specialty to be practiced only by professionally trained persons. While pastoral expertise and guidance is critical in a medical context, there are too many circumstances in which chaplaincy services are not available and a doctor or nurse may be the only one immediately available to provide spiritual support.

Many continue to conceptualize medicine as a moral and spiritual practice because it was formed by moral and spiritual communities (MacIntyre 1977,

2007). The practice of Hippocratic and Western medicine grew from a tradition in which practitioners swore oaths to divine authorities. Sacred narratives that guide many spiritual communities continue to shape the meaning and goals of medicine (Verhey 1998, 2003). When medicine is understood within a spiritual and moral framework, Curlin and Hall have argued that physicians are moral and spiritual "friends" to the sick and engage patients with wisdom, respect, and candor. They suggest that this contrasts with a conventional model of "strangers," whose relationship is characterized instead by competence, autonomy, and neutrality (Curlin and Hall 2005a).

The difference between the two models is instructive. The friendship model is influenced by the Jewish and Christian exhortation to "make friends with the physician"—the best translation of Sirach 38:15 (Skehan and Di Lella 1987). The stranger model is shaped by contemporary social dynamics such as bureaucratization, urbanization, technology, and the secularization of the public square. Advocates of the friendship model, however, see no compelling reason why these social forces demand a recharacterization of the profession unhinged from religious influences. The friendship model is grounded in a longstanding tradition of medical practice, influenced by community traditions and sacred texts, and can continue to be wisely embodied in a complex, pluralistic society.

Critics who locate the profession under contemporary norms believe that physicians are bound to a constitutional separation of church and state as is found in the case of public school educators (Scheurich 2005). This comparison does not account, however, for how physicians are a self-regulating profession and for the way that the doctor-patient relationship is legally classified under protected privacy and confidentiality laws (Annas, Glantz, and Mariner 1990). Consequently, with the exception of tort law, the patient-physician relationship is not under direct state regulation, despite federal funding. The U.S. legal framework allows for a tradition-oriented approach to medicine in which physicians consciously shape patient care through a practice influenced by their faith or worldview.

While there will continue to be diverse and competing understandings of the profession in its relationship to state and religious influences, a mitigating approach calls for an "open pluralism" by which the profession allows for differences between worldviews not requiring uniformity toward spiritual or moral questions (Kinghorn et al. 2007). Under these conditions, some physicians may engage patients on spiritual and religious issues connected to health and participate in spiritual practices such as prayer if it is discerned to be appropriate to the situation and is agreed to by the patient. Who initiates is important, and physician assessment of the many conditions that dictate the appropriateness of spiritual care in the clinical encounter is paramount (Koenig 2007).

Engagement of religion and spirituality requires practical wisdom and training rather than reliance on professional codes, which by definition lack subtlety in discerning the specifics of each case. Some physicians may not feel comfortable engaging spiritual or moral issues for personal reasons. For example, a physician may feel that it would be inauthentic to pray with a patient when he or she does not practice prayer personally. In a friendship model, physicians in such a position might honestly disclose to the patient their reasons for discomfort and suggest agreeable alternatives such as inviting a chaplain or having the patient lead in prayer while the physician passively participates. Conflict can also arise when a patient and a physician do not share the same religious faith. Some physicians and patients may not feel comfortable engaging in spiritual conversations or practices when the relationship lacks a similar belief structure. Physicians should neither conveniently avoid religion nor be required to directly participate in a religious belief or practice that is unshared. Each situation should be decided on a case-by-case basis between the physician and patient.

As candor replaces what Curlin and Hall (2005a) describe as neutrality, some patients may begin to realize how worldviews shape and alter the practice of medicine. Some patients will likely seek out physicians or institutions that share their specific values or beliefs (Curlin and Hall 2005b). Others will seek to navigate differences that put neither the patient nor the practitioner in an uncomfortable position. This moral and spiritual diversity, rather than harming the unity of the biomedical profession, will enrich its practice by allowing both patients and physicians to be more authentic, honest, and whole in the medical encounter.

Con 3: Provision of Spiritual Care Is outside the Boundaries of the Physician's Role

By the middle of the last century, paternalistic abuses and the emerging doctrine of informed consent had contributed to a consensus among bioethicists on the value of patient autonomy. Physicians increasingly recognized patients as partners in making clinical decisions affecting their welfare. At the same time, professionals in several disciplines began to question and to cross the boundaries of their disciplines: religious leaders delved into psychology, chaplains into the meeting of a variety of patient needs, and physicians into the provision of spiritual care. The ideals of holistic practice, supported by these developments and by the mandates of regulatory bodies, have contributed to the current climate in which failure to address the nonmedical aspects of people's lives could become construed as neglect.

These developments call for careful attention to the goals of medicine and to the boundaries of the physician's role. If the goal of medicine is to restore and promote health, what are the limits of health? Should health encompass spiritual health, and if so is an instrumentalist approach to spirituality by physicians justifiable? Shuman and Meador (2002), among others, argue that promoting faith for its health benefits distorts its essence.

Richard Sloan and his coauthors emphasize the ethical risks for physicians of encouraging religious activities because of their health benefits, or because they provide comfort:

> Physicians have considerable influence, which presumably derives from their medical expertise, and patients often regard their recommendations as authoritative. For example, the recommendation that a patient with pneumonia take antibiotics and restrict his or her activity is likely to be followed because the patient accepts the physician's authority. The same influence is exerted when a physician inquires about or recommends religious activities. Physicians and patients alike are on dangerous ground if they believe that advice about religious matters has the same medical support as a recommendation for antibiotic treatment. Such assumptions can have a coercive effect, and they raise ethical questions about patients' autonomy in matters of religion. (Sloan et al. 2000, p. 1914)

These authors further point out that physicians are not trained to carry out in-depth spiritual conversations with patients, and they suggest that patients are more appropriately referred to professional chaplains, who are.

Physicians who invite patients to prayer risk introducing many hidden messages to the patient that may either be detrimental or helpful. Introducing a theologically directed prayer for the agnostic or atheist may be construed as vacuous or even as an emotional assault that could affect the patient-doctor relationship, even if it is intended to demonstrate a physician's compassion. Beliefs differ, and it is usually best to enable the patient to identify and set the parameters for what will bring him greater spiritual, psychological, and emotional equanimity. Although polls indicate that not all patients would be comfortable with their physicians entering their spiritual lives, it is appropriate to inquire of patients whether they wish their doctors to acknowledge this component of their lives.

Pro 4: Physicians Should Be Allowed to Refuse Care on the Basis of Conscience

The medical profession is not a monolithic moral practice but includes individuals who hold diverse and at times incommensurate worldviews, spiritual beliefs, and viewpoints regarding the purpose and ends of medicine. There have always been diverse and sometimes rival understandings of health, disease, and healing. For example, Asclepian cults and Christian healing embedded similar Hippocratic practices in radically different worldviews, institutions, and accompanying spiritual rites (Edelstein and Edelstein 1945). Seen from a wide lens, rivalrous diversity also exists in the contemporary world when we compare modern biomedicine with alternative theories of healing such as Shamanism or traditional Chinese medicine. Within the practice of biomedicine itself, there is a growing diversity of opinion about the proper use and purposes of emerging medical technology.

Some ethicists argue that the existence of moral pluralism demands that the medical profession embrace a pluralistic practice of medicine which does not prescribe uniformity in its application of technology (Curlin and Hall 2005a). Despite irreconcilable moral diversity, it should not be concluded that biomedicine will fracture into disparate groups of healing methods and beliefs. Instead, biomedicine will continue to experience significant harmony because different moral traditions continue to agree on many aspects of the ends of medicine. Moreover, the methods and language offered by empirical science will continue to create substantial common ground uniting the profession despite irreconcilable moral differences. The profession should self-regulate its members only on those moral questions having widespread agreement within the profession and within society at large—leaving space for moral difference when no consensus can be reached.

The issue of physician conscientious objection should be conceptualized within this wider framework of moral and spiritual pluralism, and it remains a key component guiding a diverse society. Under this vision, it is axiomatic that physicians practice medicine commensurate with their worldview, spiritual communities, and personal consciences. In contrast, under the current social and political framework, rival positions attempt to construct hegemony by forcing their own moral viewpoints on the practice of everyone else—which may include constraint or compulsion on personal conscience. This process inevitably leads to an appeal to political and legal means of redress and may result in strong worry concerning the direction of the profession (Davenport 2009), questionable accusations such as selfishness (Cantor 2009), or a call for outright removal of others from the profession of medicine (Savulescu 2006). Underneath each of these accounts lies an aim of moral hegemony within medicine. But as Diana Eck has argued, "The challenge of pluralism is not to obliterate or erase difference, nor to smooth out differences under a universalizing canopy, but rather to discover ways of living, connecting, relating, arguing, and disagreeing in a society of differences" (Eck 2007, p. 745).

Living in a civil society with a cacophony of moral beliefs and practices requires deference for individual conscience, as Sulmasy emphasizes: "Respect for conscience is at the root of the concept of tolerance" (2008, p. 145). However, if we fail to allow the free exercise of conscience in the practice of medicine, then all of us, both conservative and liberal, place our consciences at risk of the whims of political control and power. In the 1966 film, *A Man for All Seasons*, the character Sir Thomas More, the 16th-century lord chancellor of England, made the acclaimed statement, "I'd give the Devil benefit of law for my own safety's sake!" While our contemporary context is different, the basic principle remains germane: to protect one's own conscience, social structures must be constructed and followed in order to protect every conscience, even those consciences which are counted immoral. The risk of harm to conscientious practice in medicine is not worth momentary political control that changes with the wind. An alternative proposal of an "open pluralism" (Kinghorn et al. 2007) bypasses the stratagem of winners and losers and creates a civic sphere in which rival moral visions and practices coexist under one professional guild.

There are two tradeoffs in following a vision of moral pluralism in the medical profession. The first is that those who hold current political power would lose legal control over certain medical technologies. Medical issues such as abortion and euthanasia would be depoliticized by creating a social framework in which individuals were free to follow a practice dictated by conscience. Physicians who desire to offer these technologies based on their worldview would be legally free. Those physicians who on moral grounds do not believe that these technologies fall under the auspices of health or healing would also be free to follow a practice guided by their moral compass. The second tradeoff is that patients would not necessarily have access to certain types of desired medical technologies. Rather than forcing physicians to provide contested technologies which violate conscience, this responsibility would be absorbed by two groups. Patients would be responsible to seek out locales where they could receive the medical technologies that they have identified as important. It is unreasonable for a patient who lives in a rural area to expect contested medical technologies to be made universally available by society; he or she might have to seek treatment outside the local area. This responsibility would also fall on advocates who value controversial types of medical technologies. They would need to create organizations aimed at identifying populations who do not have access to those medical technologies and recruit medical providers to work in those locales.

Con 4: Physicians Should Not Be Allowed to Refuse Care on the Basis of Conscience

Religious institutions such as Roman Catholic hospitals often restrict access to certain "sensitive" modes of care, including abortion, family planning, HIV counseling, infertility treatment, and termination of life support. Yet most of these institutions recognize the right of patients to obtain legal treatments, even if their providers find them morally troubling on religious or other personal grounds (White 1999). A provider may also have a right to refuse providing a treatment that he considers wrong, but does this extend to refusing to provide information about the intervention or refusing a referral to another potential source of the treatment?

The policy of the American Medical Association articulates this fundamental obligation of the physician to provide informed consent: "The patient has the right to receive information from physicians and to discuss the benefits, risks, and costs of appropriate treatment alternatives" (AMA 1993). The ethical rationale for fully informing patients is that, as the model of the physician-patient relationship shifts from paternalism toward a greater emphasis on patient autonomy, open discussion with patients both of the options available and of the physician's beliefs and recommendations is increasingly recognized as important to enhancing patients' functional autonomy. Quill and Brody (1996) contend that this means a physician needs to inform a patient if her chosen course violates the physician's fundamental values, and perhaps help the patient find another physician.

In a study of controversial clinical practices associated with religious beliefs, Curlin et al. (2007) found that many physicians would refuse to tell patients about all of their legal treatment options in several situations. The recommendation of these authors is that patients discuss these issues with their physicians in advance and, if necessary, change physicians. However, critics of this solution such as Stotland et al. (2007) respond that it is "unrealistic and unfair to expect patients to anticipate all conditions that may befall them, identify which ones might be problematic for their physicians, and agree either to reach a compromise or to seek care elsewhere." These writers point out that medical visits are typically short and focused on current needs, and that many patients are unable to change physicians. Put another way, the right of patients to legally available treatments is meaningless in the absence of physicians available to provide them.

Pro 5: Spiritual Interventions and Practices Belong in Medicine

Several spiritually based approaches are now part of mainstream practice in Western medicine. Prominent examples are twelve-step spirituality in the treatment of addictive disorders; mindfulness meditation in the treatment of conditions ranging from anxiety to personality disorders; and the relief of spiritual distress in care at the end of life. Many others, including forgiveness-based treatment and spiritually integrated psychotherapy, are accruing an evidence base, while still others are used as complementary or alternative therapies.

Reluctance to accept spiritual approaches and interventions has often been couched in scientific terms. However, scientific investigation has never been objective in the manner in which Enlightenment thinkers conceptualized or portrayed it (Polanyi 1983; Kuhn 1970). After the Enlightenment, physicians allied themselves with a scientific medicine chiefly characterized by a belief in a mind-body dualism, an ontological view of disease origin, and an emphasis on numerical measurements and probabilistic reasoning (Risse 1997). Scientific medicine portrayed itself as a profession that was objective, free from religious quackery, and authoritative (Starr 1982). This alliance has produced both a monopoly in offering health care and unprecedented social confidence.

With the rise of postmodernism, however, there has been growing insight that there is no neutral standpoint by which a physician might practice medicine in relation to spirituality, morality, or theological issues (Hall and Curlin 2004). The practice of medicine always embodies certain values and aims in which a physician finds guidance when offering medical diagnosis and treatment. Those goods and aims are inevitably undergirded by metaphysical and spiritual worldviews (MacIntyre 1990). Even something as commonplace as a physician's persuading a patient to stop smoking is in actuality grounded in certain unsubstantiated and nonempirical assumptions about the goods and aims of human life. Whenever it is presupposed that a healthy, longer life is better than something else and consequently should be pursued, there are inevitably embedded theological and religious assumptions. On what grounds can someone argue that living longer is better than living less? On what basis can it be argued that living pain-free is better than being in pain? Or more generally, why is life better than death?

These philosophical questions are directly related to the practice of medicine but cannot be answered on empirical grounds. Because one's assumptions on such basic issues are usually so unconsciously accepted, it is often difficult to see the underlying spiritual framework infused in something so simple as encouraging a patient to cease smoking. Objective data cannot in themselves ground the conclusion that a patient should stop smoking. Rather, it is a person's foundational beliefs about the meaning and purposes of human life that give meaning to the data being analyzed. These deep convictions depend on normative sources of human understanding such as theology, philosophy, and metaphysics. The manner in which human knowledge is formulated (i.e., epistemology) requires that physicians consciously acknowledge that the practice of medicine presupposes and depends on a larger theoretical framework derived from nonscientific sources (Newbigin 1986). Moreover, it calls for physicians to recognize that the nonmaterial dimensions of humanity are inherent in every patient encounter because they underlie the basic assumptions and aims of physical caring and curing (Sulmasy 1999a, 2006).

If it is true that spirituality cannot be removed from how physicians engage patients, what are the implications for potential abuse of physician authority? Some argue that spirituality should be excluded from the patient relationship because clinicians may misuse their powerful position to unduly influence patient spirituality (Sloan et al. 2000). While this may occasionally be a danger, a more substantial misuse of physician authority occurs when physicians conceptualize themselves as morally and spiritual neutral, when their counsel and care are in fact unconsciously functioning within a theologically latent worldview. A clinician's worldview manifests itself not only in what he or she actively recommends, but also on those topics in which a physician remains silent. When clinicians do not integrate spirituality into their care plan, this reflects a belief that religion and spirituality are not particularly relevant to the medical issues facing a patient (Curlin and Hall 2005a).

In this way, silence reflects a worldview that relegates religion and spirituality to a sphere of subjective values that are secondary to objective facts. But this viewpoint is itself an unsubstantiated claim about the nature of reality (Newbigin 1986). When a physician applies this construct to the doctor-patient relationship, he or she in actuality presents a particular worldview on the patient. The so-called neutral physician asserts his or her spiritual framework to patients as much as an overtly religious clinician does—but the secular context often masks these dynamics. Consequently, patients are in greater danger of moral or spiritual manipulation from "neutral" physicians because they have not been properly informed of how the clinician's worldview operates in medical decision making or care patterns. Silence toward spirituality in the medical encounter does not avoid the asymmetry of physician authority, but conceals its power. Patients are better protected through physician candor than through the appearance of neutrality.

In addition, the silence has an impact beyond the physician-patient relationship. The medical team—which may include nurses, nutritionists, social workers, and chaplains—may be integrating spiritual interventions into their practice to provide total care of the patient. The physician has an overarching ethical responsibility to be aware of and bring clarity and not ambiguity in the care of the patient. The silence can have an impact on an entire heath care setting. One medical chief walked into a conference room and quickly apologized for interrupting what he thought was a CPR class. In fact, it was a Reiki training program for medical staff. The medical chief was not aware that the practice was being offered or whether it was a spiritual practice.

Con 5: Spiritual Interventions and Practices Do Not Belong in Medicine

Physicians and patients have diverse views regarding spirituality, which remains difficult to clearly define (Bessinger and Kuhne 2002; Bregman 2004). This lack of agreement on an operational definition of spirituality suggests that physicians should proceed with caution in engaging this aspect of their patients' lives. While an atheist may feel comfortable attempting to foster a spirituality that seems psychologically beneficial to his patient, a religious believer may find this instrumental use of religion empty and ethically questionable. He would probably find even more troubling the discouragement by a secular physician of a patient's faith on the grounds that it is injurious to his health. Conversely, a religious physician's efforts to bolster his patient's faith because he believes a connection with a transcendent God is what the patient most needs could be seen as proselytizing that is inappropriate in a secular context.

Physicians should respect their patients' autonomy and, cognizant of the authority that inheres in their professional roles, avoid exerting undue influence on vulnerable patients who come to them for their medical rather than for their spiritual expertise. As Richard Sloan argues in *Blind Faith: The Unholy Alliance of Religion and Medicine* (2008), they should defer and refer spiritual interventions to those professionals with appropriate training, standards, and experience. Exceptions to this general rule should be made with close attention to informed consent, including disclosure of the clinician's worldview.

Additionally, physicians should respect their patients' privacy. As Sloan and his associates put it, "Marital status is associated with health, but physicians do not dispense advice regarding marriage" (2000, p. 1914).

Finally, the instrumental use of spiritual practices such as integrative therapies raises a number of troubling ethical questions which touch on informed consent, truth telling, and fidelity, to mention a few (Moczynski, Haker, and Bentele 2009). Physicians need to respect the cultural and religious values of patients in their care. Patients have the right to be fully informed of interventions, including spiritual practices. Spiritual practices that are offered outside of a patient's beliefs without consent can cause ambiguity, worry, and fear. Many spiritual practices overlap with secular practices such as meditation. How can patients distinguish whether the meditation practice that they are being offered at their cancer center (Reiki or other) is directed toward their spiritual or their physical healing? Can spiritual interventions ever be really separated from the traditions in which they are based? The physician needs to be truthful about the benefits and limitations of the interventions, but how can one measure or predict the benefits and limitations of a spiritual practice? There can be a blurring of professional roles in the instrumental use of spiritual practices that can erode fidelity. Is the physician also the chaplain for the patient? As one patient stated, "I wish my physician would spend less time praying for me and more time reading my CAT scan." These ethical issues involve all the members of the medical team, including the chaplain.

Conclusion

We have considered here deeply held differences regarding the role of spirituality in the physician-patient relationship. To navigate these difficult waters, physicians must bring to this relationship a knowledge of both their own and their patients' spiritualities as well as ethical sensitivity.

REFERENCES

AMA (American Medical Association). 1993. *AMA Policy E-10.01: Fundamental Elements of the Patient-Physician Relationship*. Issued June 1992; adopted June 1990 (*JAMA* 262: 33); updated 1993. Chicago: American Medical Association.

American Board of Internal Medicine. 2002. Medical professionalism in the new millennium: A physician charter. A project of the American Board of Internal Medicine Foundation ACoP-ASoIMF, European Foundation of Internal Medicine. *Annals of Internal Medicine* 136:243–46.

Annas, G. J., L. H. Glantz, and W. K. Mariner. 1990. The right of privacy protects the doctor-patient relationship. *JAMA* 263:858–61.

Balboni, M. J., and T. A. Balboni. 2010. Reintegrating care for the dying, body and soul. *Harvard Theological Review* 103:351–64.

Balboni, T. A., M. E. Paulk, M. J. Balboni, A. C. Phelps, E. T. Loggers, A. A. Wright, S. D. Block, E. F. Lewis, J. R. Peteet, and H. G. Prigerson. 2010. Provision of spiritual care to patients with advanced cancer: Associations with medical care and quality of life near death. *Journal of Clinical Oncology* 28:445–52.

Bessinger, D., and T. Kuhne. 2002. Medical spirituality: Defining domains and boundaries. *Southern Medical Journal* 95:1385–88.

Blackshaw, S. L., and J. B. Miller. 1994. Boundaries in clinical psychiatry. *American Journal of Psychiatry* 151:2.

Bregman, L. 2004. Defining spirituality: Multiple uses and murky meanings of an incredibly popular term (editorial). *Journal of Pastoral Care and Counseling* 58:157–67.

Cantor, J. D. 2009. Conscientious objection gone awry: Restoring selfless professionalism in medicine. *New England Journal of Medicine* 360:1484–85.

Charles, S. C., J. R. Wilbert, and K. J. Franke. 1985. Sued and nonsued physicians' self-reported reactions to malpractice litigation. *American Journal of Psychiatry* 142: 437–40.

Coller, B. S., P. Klotman, and L. G. Smith. 2002. Professing and living the oath: Teaching medicine as a profession. *American Journal of Medicine* 112:744–48.

Coulehan, J. 2005. Viewpoint: Today's professionalism; Engaging the mind but not the heart. *Academic Medicine* 80:892–98.

Curlin, F. A. 2008. Commentary: A case for studying the relationship between religion and the practice of medicine. *Academic Medicine* 83:1118–20.

Curlin, F. A., and D. E. Hall. 2005a. Strangers or friends? A proposal for a new spirituality-in-medicine ethic. *Journal of General and Internal Medicine* 20:370–74.

———. 2005b. Red medicine, blue medicine: Pluralism and the future of healthcare. Martin Marty Center for the Advanced Study of Religion, Religion and Culture Web Forum. May. http://divinity.uchicago.edu/martycenter/publications/webforum/052005/commentary.shtm. Accessed 5 May 2009.

Curlin, F. A., R. E. Lawrence, M. H. Chin, and J. D. Lantos. 2007. Religion, conscience, and controversial clinical practices. *New England Journal of Medicine* 356:593–600.

Davenport, M. L. 2009. Extinguishing physician conscience. *American Thinker*, 3 March. http://www.americanthinker.com/2009/03/extinguishing_physician_consci.html. Accessed 5 May 2009.

Dawkins, R. 2006. *The God Delusion*. New York: Houghton Mifflin.

Eck, D. L. 2007. Prospects for pluralism: Voice and vision in the study of religion. *Journal of the American Academy of Religion* 75:743–76.

Edelstein, E. J., and L. Edelstein. 1945. *Asclepius: A Collection and Interpretation of the Testimonies*. Baltimore: Johns Hopkins University Press.

Freidson, E. 2001. *Professionalism, the Third Logic: On the Practice of Knowledge*. Chicago: The University of Chicago Press.

Griffith, C. H., and J. F. Wilson. 2003. The loss of idealism throughout internship. *Evaluation of Health Professions* 26:415–26.

Gutheil, T. G., and G. O. Gabbard. 1993. The concept of boundaries in clinical practice: Theoretical and risk-management dimensions. *American Journal of Psychiatry* 150: 188–96.

Hall, D. E., and F. A. Curlin. 2004. Can physicians' care be neutral regarding religion? *Academic Medicine* 79:677–79.

Hippocratic Registry. 2008. *Hippocratic Registry International.* Available at http://hippocraticregistry.com/OathspledgesMor1.html. Accessed 22 May 2009.

Hitchens, C. 2007. *God Is Not Great: How Religion Poisons Everything*. New York: Hachette Book Group.

Huddle, T. S. 2005. Viewpoint: Teaching professionalism; Is medical morality a competency? *Academic Medicine* 80:885–91.

Jonsen, A. R. 1983. Watching the doctor. *New England Journal of Medicine* 308:1531–35.

Kinghorn, W. A., M. D. McEvoy, A. Michel, and M. Balboni. 2007. Professionalism in modern medicine: Does the emperor have any clothes? *Academic Medicine* 82:40–45.

Koenig, H. G. 2007. *Spirituality in Patient Care: Why, How, When, and What*. Rev. 2nd ed. Philadelphia: Templeton Foundation Press.

Kuhn, T. S. 1970. *The Structure of Scientific Revolutions,* 2nd ed. Chicago: University of Chicago Press.

Larkin, G. L., M. P. McKay, and P. Angelos. 2005. Six core competencies and seven deadly sins: A virtues-based approach to the new guidelines for graduate medical education. *Surgery* 138:490–97.

Lind, G. 2000. Moral regression in medical students and their learning environment. *Revista Brasileira de Educacao Medica* 24, no. 3: 24–33.

Lo, B., D. Ruston, L. W. Kates, R. M. Arnold, C. B. Cohen, K. Faber-Langendoen, S. Z. Pantilat, et al. 2002. Discussing religious and spiritual issues at the end of life: A practical guide for physicians. *JAMA* 287:749–54.

MacIntyre, A. C. 1977. Patients as agents. In *Philosophical Medical Ethics: Its Nature and Significance*, ed. H. T. Engelhardt and S. F. Spicker. Dordrecht: Reidel.

———. 1990. *Three Rival Versions of Moral Enquiry: Encyclopaedia, Genealogy, and Tradition*. Gifford Lectures delivered at the University of Edinburgh, 1988. Notre Dame, IN: University of Notre Dame Press.

———. 2007. *After Virtue: A Study in Moral Theory*. 3rd ed. Notre Dame, IN: University of Notre Dame Press.

Massachusetts Board. 1994. *General Guidelines Related to the Maintenance of Boundaries in the Practice of Psychotherapy by Physicians (Adult Patients)*. Boston: Massachusetts Board of Registration in Medicine.

Medical Oaths. 2009. Timeline for Medical Oaths, 600 BC–2009. Google search for "medical oaths." www.google.com. Accessed 22 May 2009.

Minkler, M. 2005. *Community Organizing and Community Building for Health*. 2nd ed. New Brunswick, NJ: Rutgers University Press.

Moczynski, W., H. Haker, and K. Bentele, eds. 2009. *Medical Ethics in Health Care Chaplaincy*. Berlin: Lit Verlag.

Newbigin, L. 1986. *Foolishness to the Greeks: The Gospel and Western Culture*. Grand Rapids, MI: Eerdmans.

Pal, A. 2006. The Dalai Lama interview. *The Progressive*, January. www.progressive.org/mag_intv0106. Accessed 18 Jan. 2010.

Polanyi, M. 1983. *The Tacit Dimension*. Gloucester, MA: Peter Smith.

Puchalski, C. M. 2008. Addressing the spiritual needs of patients. *Cancer Treatment Research* 140:79–91.

Quill, T. E., and H. Brody. 1996. Physician recommendations and patient autonomy: Finding a balance between physician power and patient choice. *Annals of Internal Medicine* 125:763–69.

Risse, G. B. 1997. Medical care. In *Companion Encyclopedia of the History of Medicine*, ed. W. F. Bynum and R. Porter. London: Routledge.

Savulescu, J. 2006. Conscientious objection in medicine. *British Medical Journal* 332: 294–97.

Scheurich, N. 2003. Reconsidering spirituality and medicine. *Academic Medicine* 78:356–60.

———. 2005. Spirituality, medicine, and the possibility of wisdom. *Journal of General and Internal Medicine* 20:379–80.

Shuman. J. J., and K. G. Meador. 2002. *Heal Thyself: Spirituality, Medicine and the Distortion of Christianity*. New York: Oxford University Press.

Shanafelt, T. D., K. A. Bradley, J. F. Wipf, and A. L. Back. 2002. Burnout and self-reported patient care in an internal medicine residency program. *Annals of Internal Medicine* 136:358–67.

Sinnott-Armstrong, W. 2009. *Morality without God?* New York: Oxford University Press.

Skehan, P. W., and A. A. Di Lella. 1987. *The Wisdom of Ben Sira: A New Translation with Notes*. Garden City, NY: Doubleday.

Sloan, R. P. 2008. *Blind Faith: The Unholy Alliance of Religion and Medicine*. New York: St. Martin's.

Sloan, R. P., E. Bagiella, L. VandeCreek, M. Hover, C. Casalone, T. Jinpu Hirsch, Y. Hasan,

R. Kreger, and P. Poulos. 2000. Should physicians prescribe religious activities? *New England Journal of Medicine* 342:1913–16.
Smith, D. C. 1996. The Hippocratic Oath and modern medicine. *Journal of Historical Medicine and Allied Science* 51:484–500.
Starr, P. 1982. *The Social Transformation of American Medicine.* New York: Basic Books.
Stenger, V. J. 2007. *God: The Failed Hypothesis; How Science Shows That God Does Not Exist.* New York: Prometheus Books.
Stotland, N. L., L. F. Ross, E. W. Clayton, J. Z. Mishtal, W. Chavkin, V. Zarate, P. O'Connell, et al. 2007. Religion, conscience, and controversial clinical practices. *New England Journal of Medicine* 356:1889–92.
Sulmasy, D. P. 1999a. Is medicine a spiritual practice? *Academic Medicine* 74:1002–5.
———. 1999b. What is an oath and why should a physician swear one? *Theoretical Medicine and Bioethics* 20:329–46.
———. 2002. A biopsychosocial-spiritual model for the care of patients at the end of life. *Gerontologist* 42:24–33.
———. 2006. *The Rebirth of the Clinic: An Introduction to Spirituality in Health Care.* Washington, DC: Georgetown University Press.
———. 2008. What is conscience and why is respect for it so important? *Theoretical Medicine and Bioethics* 29:135–49.
Verhey, A. 1998. The doctor's oath—and a Christian swearing it. In *On Moral Medicine*, ed. S. E. Lammers and A. Verhey. Grand Rapids, MI: Eerdmans.
———. 2003. *Reading the Bible in the Strange World of Medicine.* Grand Rapids, MI: Eerdmans.
White, K. A. 1999. Crisis of conscience: Reconciling religious faith care providers' beliefs and patients' rights. *Stanford Law Review* 51:1703–50.
Zuckerman, P. 2008. *Society without God: What the Least Religious Nations Can Tell Us about Contentment.* New York: New York University Press.

CHAPTER THIRTEEN

Spiritual Care and Chaplaincy

Terry R. Bard, D.D., and
Walter Moczynski, D.Min., M.T.S., M.Div.

The earliest human records document provisions for spiritual and religious care. Health and well-being have been intimately intertwined throughout history, often in communal life and frequently in religious belief and practices. Religious leaders were originally the arbiters of practices directed to address both physical and spiritual well-being, and religious beliefs and forms provided the contexts for undergirding this relationship. Whereas most early cultures shared the perspective that body, mind, and spirit were integrated functions, and believed that problems occurring in any one of these three dimensions affected the other two, Greek culture offered a different conception of the relationship, suggesting that body, mind, and spirit each had its own independent integrity and reality. Greek notions took hold in the Middle East and influenced early Christianity. In ancient cultures the concept of *soma sema*, the body as the prison of the spirit (or "soul"), became embedded in both theory and practice as formal disciplines relating to these dimensions emerged. The priest or shaman, formerly arbiter of all three, emerged as the communal overseer of the spirit, while the physician became the caretaker of the body, and the philosopher addressed the concerns of the mind.

Over the centuries, societies and individuals have struggled to relate these three aspects of human experience. A number of debates during the early 20th century left most Western professional practitioners with the belief that these realms, though sharing some overlapping concerns, were independent of each other. Physicians were to concern themselves with bodily things; the newly emerging practitioners of psychology, neurology, and psychiatry were to address the mind; and religious leaders were to devote their efforts to the spirit. Exceptions such as Christian Science notwithstanding, the dominant model for Western society was a separatist one.

Challenges to this separatist model persisted, however. Alternative practices emerged in the 1960s and early 1970s, as Anglican bishop John Robinson and others declared God dead, as experimental psychology evolved into clinical psychology, and as medicine began to learn of relationships among body, stress, and belief. The early 21st-century reconsideration of the relationship of body, mind, and spirit may sort out differently than it did a century ago.

Pastoral care occurred informally and haphazardly in hospital settings before the 20th century. Most frequently it occurred through the administration of religious rites and sacraments by clergy. A number of cultures and religious traditions regarded visiting the sick as a special obligation of their membership or their clerical representatives. More focused education in clinical pastoral care began during the early 20th century coincident with ongoing formal debates over the relationship between religion and medicine. Richard Clark Cabot, M.D. (1869–1939), frequently credited as one of the founders of the pastoral education movement, began working with ministerial students at Worcester State Hospital. One of his students, Anton T. Boisen, later became a patient at the same institution. During his hospitalization and eventual recovery, Boisen began to appreciate the analytical approach to care that he had experienced. He concluded that such an approach, which used objective assessment and knowledge of human predicaments as a template, would benefit ministers in their pastoral function. Boisen posited that all individuals were "living human documents" who need to be understood and ministered to in this context.

The suggestion of such early pioneers that the pastor, too, should engage in self-reflection as a living human document marked the beginning of what has come to be known as clinical pastoral education (CPE). This movement evolved over time to become a model for training. Initially, Protestant "pastors" were trained; by the 1990s ordained clergy of many denominations sought proficiency in clinical skills, team work, and self-reflection. More recently, such training has also become available for many nonclergy who express interest in providing pastoral and spiritual care. All professional pastoral care organizations today require candidates seeking board certification to have successfully completed a minimum of four CPE "units" comprising 400 hours each of a mixture of didactic, interactive, and supervisory experiences.

Clinical pastoral training that originally took place in hospitals expanded to a broad range of institutional and organizational training sites, and collaboration with Protestant seminaries helped to provide an academic structure. Eventually offering a variety of training levels along with a coterie of advanced, experienced trainers, CPE educators created an association for collaboration, strengthening, and standardization—the Association for Clinical Pastoral Education (ACPE). ACPE remains the largest CPE association but has spawned at least two alternative models, the College of Pastoral Supervision and Psychotherapy (CPSP) and the Catholic Model. These nationally accredited CPE programs are both competitive and collaborative and, together, oversee CPE training.

Although CPE was initially designed to help pastors function more effectively in parish settings, this new training effort provided ministers with skills compatible with the medical model which they could use in the medical settings where their training had taken place. A new emphasis on CPE led to the creation of the professional hospital chaplain along with organizational structures to board-certify chaplains. Formerly, religious ordination was considered sufficient for such offices, and clergy presence was often limited to matters relating to trauma and death, usually focused on religious rites. With the emergence of CPE a number of mostly urban hospitals began to create formal departments of pastoral care, and it became common for clergy to be available to patients. By the 1960s, this growth extended well beyond the acute care setting and into nursing and rehabilitation centers, psychiatric institutions, prisons, and eventually into businesses and the community at large.

Groups of individuals trained in clinical pastoral care formed their own associations relating to the kind of settings in which they functioned—for example, associations of prison chaplains, mental health chaplains, acute care chaplains, nursing home chaplains, community chaplains, and business and industrial chaplains among others. While most clergy trained were Protestant, in the late 1960s and 1970s these associations began to accept trained religious leaders from non-Protestant backgrounds. Catholics created their own association in the mid-1960s, and Jewish-trained rabbis and cantors created their own in the 1980s.

Each of these associations, whether defined by functional setting or religious affiliation, provided both a social and professional home for CPE (or equivalently trained) chaplains. Formalized structures to professionalize membership by providing board certification proliferated with the endorsement of health care chaplaincy in the 1980s by the Joint Commission on Accreditation of Hospitals (JCAH), the predecessor of the current JCAHO—the Joint Commission on Accreditation of Healthcare Organizations. Currently, it is not uncommon for Catholic and Jewish chaplains to receive board certification both from the organization representing their institutional setting and from that representing their religious faith.

In the 1970s, the ACPE determined that it would expand its educational programs to include lay people in addition to seminary students and ordained or invested clergy. This effort has expanded greatly and now includes programs focused on training doctors, nurses, and others from a variety of health care disciplines.

Chaplaincy today reflects a number of other societal shifts begun in the 1960s. Challenges to authority of every kind led many to question traditional models of ordination or investiture—once considered normative for leadership and the only pathway toward religious or spiritual fulfillment and, for some, salvation. The introduction of Eastern religions and "new spirituality" meant less emphasis on fundamentals, religious history, philosophy, parochial values, and leadership. Growing attention to personal well-being, reflected in and promoted by self-psychology, contributed to the adoption of a model of chaplaincy that is more broadly inclusive, and less bound by history, tradition, and formal religious practice. Older models have not disappeared, but chaplains today come with more diverse, less clerical backgrounds. Because the expertise of the past is no longer considered necessary preparation for practice today, many come lacking any kind of formalized clinical pastoral training, but the CPE model offers the persevering the potential of becoming board certified. Whereas in the past most clergy and chaplains were male, today's chaplains are predominantly female. Some are integrated into care teams and become part of interdisciplinary care that includes attention to patients' spiritual needs. However, most continue to work in settings in which they are the designated independent providers of religious and spiritual aspects of care.

One presumption of pastoral care that remains is that all people have a spiritual, possibly even a religious, component to their lives. Pastoral caregivers aim to empower people to acknowledge and enhance this dimension. New models of CPE for certifying physicians, nurses, social workers, and others as chaplains suggest that what the traditionally religious chaplain offered was not necessarily unique, though it was honed by significant training and supervision. Whether one views the expansion of CPE to a more diverse, less "clerical" group as a dilution or as an enhancement of pastoral care, it is important to recognize the shifts in emphasis, background, and training that have taken place in many chaplains today. They may lack specific knowledge about one or many religious traditions and histories, philosophy and theology in its many varieties, and theories of personality development. When present, this background is still vital for chaplains to provide skilled counsel and support to those caring for others, enabling them to become spiritual caregivers capable of addressing an increasing number of tasks formerly relegated to the chaplain.

Many physicians who hold strong religious or spiritual beliefs acknowledge that they pray for their patients—privately, possibly after hours, or in their formal religious practices. It is increasingly common for some patients ask physicians to pray for their well-being. There are many ways for the physician to respond other than to refer such a request to the chaplain or to the patient's spiritual leader. It is usually most helpful and appropriate to invite the patient to identify the components of the prayer, possibly even to construct and state the prayer in the physician's presence as witness. Touch is often helpful at such times.

The Roles of the Chaplain and of the Physician in Providing Spiritual Care

Hospital chaplains today function in a variety of roles: as spiritual care providers for patients; as supports, resources, and consultants for the clinicians caring for them; as advisors to institutions on the design and implementation of programs and spaces to enhance spiritual life; and as members of ethics teams and committees. Here, we focus on the chaplain as a partner with the physician in the spiritual care of the patient.

Twenty-first-century physicians trained in Western medicine face many challenges in providing optimal care. Not only must they comprehend and use an abundance of resources, but also their efforts to provide expert, specialized care sometimes thwart efforts to care for their patients as whole people. Nonetheless, there is a growing consensus that care should encompass the physical, psychological, and spiritual needs of the person. As the Joint Commission, an independent accrediting and certifying organization for health care organizations, states: "The patient's beliefs and practices can affect the perception of illness and how he or she approaches treatment. Staff should accommodate the patient's unique needs whenever possible" (Joint Commission 2010, p. 21).

Patients' spiritual values constitute a connection to the world around them, a guide for purpose and meaning. These values can reflect the nature of their relationships with others, their God, or any other important dimension of their lives. The patient may nurture these values individually as well as within a religion. These values may influence patients' attitudes and behavior involving their health care—for example, in guiding patients to request a special diet or to refuse blood products.

As both medical care and spiritual care have evolved, physicians are increasingly encouraged to inquire about the relevance of their patients' spiritual values to their medical care. Many are also asking how they can ensure that their patients' spiritual and religious needs are met within the context of the doctor–patient relationship. The physician has an advocate and resource for such inquiry in the professional spiritual care provider, commonly known as the chaplain.

Chaplains offer a unique resource for spiritual and emotional care within hospitals, community clinics, and mental health centers, as well as in other settings such as schools and businesses. As suggested above, this care is not limited to patient and patient family care; it extends to physicians, medical teams, staff, and the entire health care community. Chaplains also play seminal roles as educators, enabling and guiding health care professionals to assess and offer spiritual care. Even chaplains who are educated, trained, and grounded in a religious or spiritual tradition are open to all people, including those adhering to formal religious and spiritual traditions as well as those without such backgrounds.

In their own work with patients, chaplains create time and space for the patients' stories to unfold and from these stories develop detailed plans for spiritual care. Such plans may include resources from within or outside of the care facility. The spiritual care department of a health care institution may have available chaplains representing the faith of the patient or interfaith chaplains. Patients may ask chaplains to become their primary spiritual care providers or ask them to contact a particular spiritual care provider such as an imam, rabbi, minister, or priest on their behalf through the chaplain's connections to local faith communities. Undergirding the professional chaplain-patient relationship is a code of ethics which mandates that the chaplain cannot attempt to convert patients or staff to the chaplain's spiritual or religious beliefs.

Chaplains meet and respond to patients in ways congruent with patients' beliefs. This response entails their personal presence when desired and may or may not include sharing something written, offering rites and rituals, or providing some sort of a creative response. The written word can range from sacred texts such as the Torah, the Quran, or the Bible to poetry or something written by the patient. Rites and rituals rich in meaning include blessings, prayers, or even formal services such as weddings, memorials, or namings, among others. Creative responses that enable patients to further explore their beliefs include works of art, music, or other expressions that have profound meaning to the patients.

Chaplains offer and facilitate spiritual care that addresses a wide range of concerns, such as a search for meaning and purpose; coping with grief, loss, and life crises; addressing spiritual needs; and discussing or resolving ethical dilemmas. They may offer spiritual care directly to an individual in the form of a prayer or blessing, or to a group of patients or staff—for example, at a worship or memorial service.

In their roles as teachers, chaplains can offer information and skills that open opportunities to physicians, other medical team members, and staff of the health care facility to enhance their awareness of ways to respond to the many religious and spiritual questions, beliefs, and practices of their patients. Chaplains also recognize that spiritual care is often provided by family members, friends, volunteers, and nonordained community ministers and visitors.

Spiritual concerns and attempts to address them may create tension when there is conflict between the patient's beliefs and medical treatment, among family members and friends, and among members of the medical team. Therefore, providing spiritual care is best undertaken with great caution, care, and forethought. Patients may experience distressing pressure if they conclude that someone is imposing a spiritual or religious belief on them. Reflective practice, which is increasingly taught in medical as well as pastoral care settings, can be helpful in ensuring that patients feel that they and their spiritual values are being treated with respect.

Reflective Practice: A Common Thread

Reflective practice takes many forms. In spiritual care, these include prayer, meditation, and sacred readings. Prayer is understood variously to be communication with God, deities, or, in some traditions, with the departed or with a person's own projections. Prayer can be an expression of a petition, a transfer of worry and fear, an expression of praise, or a thanksgiving. Petitionary prayer may be a cry for a physical cure or a need for forgiveness. Prayers of transfer reduce stress in situations where a patient has no control of an outcome. Prayers of praise and thanksgiving may celebrate a remission or cure or that the patient does not feel alone in his or her ordeal of illness or death. Many consider meditation and sacred readings forms of prayer.

Sharing this common thread of reflection can enable physicians and other caregivers to understand and respond respectfully to their patients. Occasionally, however, patients may invite physicians to actively engage in some sort of spiritual or religious practice such as prayer with or for them. Physicians differ in how they think they can respond to such requests in ways that both maintain professional boundaries and demonstrate respect for their patients' requests. Some physicians opt to offer a reflective response in a moment of silence, thereby respecting and honoring the request. Other physicians may decide to pray with the patient. Chaplains provide important resources to help physicians navigate such spiritual and religious requests from patients.

Sacred reflective practices are frequently important for patients who are managing acute or chronic illnesses. In a study of hospital patients, 90 percent indicated that religion was an important factor in coping with their situation (Koenig 1998), and 57 percent of Americans in a survey indicated that they believe that God can intervene to save a dying person (Jacobs, Burns, and Jacob 2008). These findings highlight that many people do not rely on medicine alone to manage their illnesses. In a 2002 survey of complementary and alternative therapy use conducted by the Centers for Disease Control and Prevention and the National Center for Health Studies, 77 percent of those surveyed indicated that prayer was the number one alternative and complementary therapy used by individuals (Barnes et al. 2004).

Reflective practices are also an important source of insight into the core of patients' spiritual identities and beliefs.

The Patient's Beliefs

Every person seeks meaning and purpose and develops a philosophy of life that addresses the age-old questions: Where did I come from? Why am I here? Where am I going? The beliefs of many people include a spiritual or religious component that addresses not only these questions, but those about healing, for example, in terms of divine intervention and miracles.

Personal beliefs are likely to evolve and transform over a lifetime. Yet they may surface only at key life events such as a birth of a child, a wedding, a divorce, serious illness, or death. Patients' past and current beliefs may have nurtured them or may have caused harm. Because of the infinite horizon of possibilities of spiritual and religious beliefs, it is critical to understand a patient's unique story in order to understand his or her spiritual and religious needs.

Asking about a patient's spiritual or religious story often begins well before the first contact with the physician. Along with basic insurance information, many hospitals and clinics ask questions about religious and spiritual preference during the admission process. This question may be simple for some to answer, but complex or embarrassing for others. A patient asked to state a religious identification may turn to a spouse and ask, "What am I?" Some patients may be afraid of being "labeled" and worry about creating a negative impact on their care or clinical outcome, even though religious and spiritual information is private, protected by Health Insurance Portability and Accountability Act (HIPAA); it cannot be released to anyone without the patient's explicit permission. Only members of the care team, which includes chaplains, have access to this information.

Once the patient's story begins to unfold, the physician is in a unique position to offer spiritual care resources to assist in his or her spiritual or religious journey. He can assure a patient who reports being grounded in his or her personal beliefs that these will be respected and that appropriate accommodation will be made throughout the patient's care. Not all patients claim to have a religious or spiritual identity on admission or when visiting their physicians; some claim to have none. On the other hand, many people are searching for a personal spiritual or religious belief and are not connected with a faith community; these patients may find themselves simultaneously in a faith crisis and a medical one.

Spiritual and religious assessment takes time and depends on patients' sense that the listener is open to hearing their stories unfold. Some chapters in these stories may reflect a desire for spiritual healing, along with hopes for physical cure.

Spiritual Healing and Cure

How can physicians deal with patients' integration of their religious and spiritual practices with their medical care and with the fact that they are searching for healing that may or may not refer to physical cure? In addition to physical healing, patients may be seeking an emotional or spiritual wholeness that enables them to be at peace with themselves and others and, possibly, to enjoy an improved relationship with God. Healing may allow one to live freely even as one is dying.

For some, however, healing represents only physical cure. The deep desire of many patients to be cured makes them vulnerable to harm from care providers unless the meaning that healing and cure have for them is clearly understood. The physician's response to patients' desires for healing can deepen the trust in the patient-physician relationship or it can inflict harm.

Attempts at spiritual care can be harmful if the patient feels that a spiritual practice will effect a physical cure. Between 1975 and 1995, 196 children in the United States died because of spiritually related medical neglect (Asser and Swan 1998). A spiritual healer may be a "faith healer," a priest or minister proclaiming special divine powers, or a member of a medical establishment. The Association of Professional Chaplains lists 40 complementary spiritual practices, such as anointing with oil, chanting, hypnosis, and Reiki (APC 2008). Practitioners include nurses, social workers, and other care providers. When seeking these practices within medical settings, patients sometimes wonder if such practices are based on science, divine intervention, or both. They can erroneously come to believe that physical cure might be possible when, in fact, it is not.

A physician can support a patient's spiritual care by monitoring the patient's understanding of the alternative and complementary practices in use during treatment, clarifying when necessary the difference between medical therapy and spiritual care. Therapies are medical practices such as conventional treatment to treat and cure an illness. Spiritual care involves the use of reflective spiritual modalities with the intention of contributing to spiritual and emotional well-being and healing. An increase in spiritual wholeness may have physical correlates and even make cure possible. However, spiritual healing is designed to bring wholeness and peace without regard to a physical cure. In most spiritual and religious traditions, God is always at work, even when cure does not take place, in the physical, emotional, and spiritual healing of a person.

Chaplains and Physicians

Increasingly, both chaplains and physicians understand the importance of a more holistic understanding of patients and strive to include important elements of patients' lives in the context of their care. Patients sometimes turn to their physicians for support and comfort, and it is not uncommon that they might request that their physician "pray for them" or offer some other "healing" remedy that is external to the physician's clinical training and expertise. Patients may also speak of their fears, wishes, beliefs, and hopes in ways that might leave physicians a bit uncomfortable. Some physicians enter these dimensions of patients' lives; others may simply refer patients to spiritual leaders or to chaplains. Chaplains can often assist the physician to enter this more amorphous arena of their patients' lives, supporting and coaching them through the process. Often, physicians who obtain such support and opt for providing a more expanded role in caring for their patients find themselves much more comfortable in entering discussions about beliefs and values with their patients.

Reasons for Caution and Optimism

Patients increasingly wish to incorporate their spiritual or religious beliefs in their approach to medical treatment. However, both caution and optimism are warranted in helping them to do so.

One reason for caution is the potential for a physician to blur professional medical boundaries. The physician who attempts to incorporate spirituality into his or her practice may find that a patient relates to him in the role of rabbi, minister, imam, or priest. What might such unsought transformations jeopardize or promote in the physician's capacity to continue providing medical care?

A physician's adoption of these roles also calls into question the accountability and responsibility of other spiritual caregivers within the medical team. Workshops or programs in spiritual care for nonchaplain caregivers provide valuable continuing education but carry potential risks. Even when care is provided in an interfaith context, it is a disservice to offer spiritual or religious care if a faith community is not available to support and endorse that care. Without the backing of a community of faith, the physician, nurse, or social worker who takes on the role of individual spiritual care provider lacks the accountability and responsibility necessary for ensuring sustainable spiritual care.

At the same time, the growing awareness that a physician can play a critical role in respecting and responding to the spiritual needs of patients is reason for optimism. The physician can begin by serving as a spiritual bridge until a professional spiritual care provider can support the patient if, after assessment, such a referral is indicated. While recalling his oath to "First, do no harm," the physician can also achieve great good by responding to the spiritual needs of the patient and creating an environment of healing and growth.

REFERENCES

APC (Association of Professional Chaplains). 2008. Complementary spiritual practices in professional chaplaincy. www.professionalchaplains.org. Accessed 16 June 2009.

Asser, S. M., and R. Swan. 1998. Child fatalities from religious-motivated medical neglect. *Journal of the American Academy of Pediatrics* 101:625–29.

Barnes, P. M., E. Powell-Griner, K. McFann, and R. L. Nahin. 2004. Complementary and alternative medicine use among adults: United States, 2002. *Advance Data from Vital and Health Statistics*, no. 343 (May 27), 1–109. www.cdc.gov/nchs/data/ad/ad343.pdf . Accessed 7 July 2009.

Jacobs, L. M., K. Burns, and B. Jacobs. 2008. Trauma death: Views of the public and trauma professionals on death and dying from injuries. *Archives of Surgery* 143:730–35.

Joint Commission. 2010. Advancing Effective Communication, Cultural Competence, and Patient- and Family-Centered Care: A Roadmap for Hospitals. www.jointcommission.org/assets/1/6/ARoadmapforHospitalsfinalversion727.pdf. Accessed 14 Mar. 2011.

Koenig, H. G. 1998. Religious attitudes and practices of hospitalized medically ill older patients. *International Journal of Psychiatry in Medicine* 49:1717–22.

CHAPTER FOURTEEN

Teaching and Learning at the Interface of Medicine and Spirituality

Marta D. Herschkopf, M.St., M.D.

As the preceding chapters indicate, interest in the traditionally important role of spirituality in medicine waned with the 20th-century development of a scientific approach to medicine and scientific dominance of the biomedical model. This chapter explores the recent resurgence of interest in spirituality in medicine, primarily at the level of medical school training.

Historically, medical school training has been a critical force in determining the type of practitioner that physicians become. Highly regulated, it institutionalizes social values and attitudes in the form of the core competencies demanded of every practicing U.S. physician. While the role of spirituality in individual practices naturally reflects personality, specialty, patient population, informal learning experiences, and other variables, there is a growing consensus that all physicians would benefit from a minimal level of what might be termed spiritual competence, to serve their patients' needs as well as possibly their own.

After reviewing 20th-century medical education and the educational reform movements that anticipated the reintroduction of spirituality, I discuss what has come to be a movement toward spirituality in medicine, identifying its supporting institutions and advocates, including Christina Puchalski, of the George Washington Institute for Spirituality and Health (GWish). I then use the historical development of the Harvard Medical School curriculum as an example of one attempt to incorporate spirituality into formal medical education, as well as the challenges encountered in doing so.

Historical Considerations

Modern U.S. medical education began with the Flexner revolution, a series of reforms that standardized admissions requirements and curricula for American medical schools. Abraham Flexner, headmaster of a private high school in the Midwest, was appointed by the Carnegie Foundation for the Advancement of Teaching to survey the contemporary state of medical education. His report, *Medical Education in the United States and Canada*, published in 1910, thrust the need for reform into the public sphere.

Flexner's report criticized the lax admissions requirements and minimal training offered by U.S. medical schools. Many schools would certify any applicant who could afford their fees as a licensed physician if the applicant merely attended a few months of lectures. Through the reforming efforts of Flexner and others, by the end of the 1920s medical schools had developed stringent admissions requirements as well as a four-year curriculum divided into preclinical and clinical years, with required instruction in basic sciences and clinical clerkship experience (Ludmerer 1999, pp. 3–6).

The first major changes to follow Flexner's revolution were a series of experimental educational programs in "comprehensive medicine" developed in the 1940s and 1950s. The corpus of medical knowledge had grown so exponentially after World War II that increasing specialization was becoming necessary to maintain competence. As a result, medical school faculties became concerned that their students were losing sight of the psychosocial and environmental factors that were as important to understanding and treating patients as the scientific details. Particularly worried that the physician-patient relationship was suffering, Cornell and the University of Colorado introduced new courses for fourth-year students in the early 1950s, and Case Western Reserve attempted a revision of its entire curriculum. These reforms emphasized environmental and preventive medicine as well as communication skills. Ultimately, however, they were discontinued because of budgetary concerns and a lack of philosophical consensus (Kendall and Reader 1988).

The next major change began in the late 1970s, when it became increasingly acknowledged that medical education in particular, and the health care system in general, had developed a number of fundamental flaws. Among these was the sense that modern mainstream medicine had, for lack of a better term, "lost its soul." While soaring costs and systemic barriers to care were part of the problem, the public also increasingly began to express dissatisfaction with the quality of the physician encounter itself. Patients felt that their doctors did not listen to them, did not understand them, and most important, seemed uninterested in them as people. Instead, doctors focused on laboratory results and procedures.

Physicians began to recognize that, despite excellent scientific training, they were often unable to satisfy their patients' concerns. Summarizing these attitudes in a 1977 article in *Science*, psychiatrist George Engel scathingly assessed the current biomedical model as "no longer adequate for the scientific tasks and social responsibilities of . . . medicine" (p. 129). As a result, patients began to turn increasingly to alternative medical approaches (Kleinman, Eisenberg, and Good 1978). At the same time, hospitals came to be perceived as cold, impersonal, and uncaring.

With hospitals no longer sacred cows and therefore no longer immune to media investigation and ridicule, the public became more aware of the shortcomings of hospital-based medical training. The infamous 1984 Libby Zion case, in which the teenage daughter of journalist Sidney Zion died from an allegedly lethal drug combination prescribed by an overworked on-call resident, dominated the headlines. It illuminated the failure of the medical training system and sparked a reform movement to curtail residents' work hours (New York Times 1987). The public began to grow concerned about the rites of passage in medical education. Reports emerged of medical students being "abused" by faculty and house staff (Silver and Glicksen 1990) and of students losing their moral compass in the high-stress environment of clinical clerkships (Feudtner, Christakis, and Christakis 1994).

The exponential expansion of graduate training programs in the second half of the century meant that supervision of medical students in the clinical rotations increasingly fell to residents, who, under impossible time pressures, would lose patience with their students as well as with their patients. Attending physicians had little sympathy for the house staff, who, in turn, had no empathy for the medical students. The prevailing attitude was: "I went through it; you can too. In fact, I had it even worse, so don't complain."

Predictably, medical students quickly learned to model their behavior on that of the often-cynical house staff with whom they spent most of their clinical training. This problem was compounded by the passage of Medicare and Medicaid in 1965, followed by the rise of managed care in the 1980s, which substantially increased the workload of physicians-in-training. Hospitals took advantage of low-paid house staff to contain their costs. Hospitals and physicians, in an effort to move patients in and out as quickly as possible, had little if any time for patients' nonmedical concerns or anything else that interfered with efficiency (Ludmerer 1999, pp. 357–62).

The drive for efficiency created a demand to "cut to the chase." This meant a growing reliance on impersonal and invasive diagnostic procedures. As early as 1932, the Commission on Medical Education noted educators' complaints about students' overreliance on laboratory tests and preoccupation with making a diagnosis to the exclusion of dealing with patients' concerns (AAMC 1932, p. 254; compare Peabody 1927). As diagnostic technology advanced, this trend increased. Furthermore, the "malpractice crisis" that began in the 1980s increased the practice of "defensive medicine," in which physicians ordered superfluous tests and procedures that they did not deem necessary, to protect themselves from litigation in the rare instance of having dismissed as benign what was in fact a grave illness. From the practitioners' perspective, it was preferable to saddle the system, and patients, with unnecessary exams rather than to suffer the devastating consequences of a missed diagnosis (McQuade 1991; Newsweek 1987). Thus developed a medical culture that valued speed and comprehensiveness but lost sight of the human factor in the clinical encounter.

By the 1990s, a variety of humanizing trends in medical education had emerged. These included the replacement of didactic lectures with problem-based learning (Neville and Norman 2007), the introduction of clinical material earlier in the curriculum (Tosteson 1990), and the imposition of legally mandated limits for "on-call" hours (Philibert, Friedmann, and Williams 2002). Two curriculum changes in particular were relevant to spirituality, as they concerned not only the acquisition of knowledge, but also the communication of values and attitudes. The first was a new emphasis on professionalism, which included ethics, communication skills, and accountability. The second was the rise of training in cultural competence, which grew out of a concern for discrepancies in access to health care for minority populations.

While the reforms of the 1940s and 1950s anticipated these trends to some extent, what was fundamentally different about the modern reforms was the focus on the moral consciousness of physicians (Kendall and Reader 1988). It had been assumed previously that such compassionate values were what drew students to the profession in the first place and that communication skills would be learned implicitly through demonstration by experienced physicians during the clerkship years. This process of unconscious patterning and implicit socialization in medical school has been termed "the hidden curriculum" and was thought to be far more powerful than any explicit didactic intervention that a school might implement (Hafferty and Franks 1994). The consensus had been that moral values could be taught only by example, not in lecture. By the 1980s, it had become unequivocally clear that the hidden curriculum had failed.

In 1981, the American Association of Medical Colleges (AAMC) created the Panel on the General Professional Education of the Physician and College Preparation for Medicine (GPEP) to consider the issue of professionalism in medical education. Its final report, published in 1984, emphasized, among other things, a shifting of emphases in medical education: "Medical faculties should emphasize the acquisition and development of skills, values, and attitudes by students at least to the same extent that they do their acquisition of knowledge." However, there was no explicit discussion in the report of what constitutes these values and attitudes, and no recommendations for how to impart them other than to "limit the amount of factual information that students are expected to memorize" (AAMC 1984, p. 1).

When a survey of programs in the early 1990s demonstrated that few medical schools had followed the recommendations of the GPEP report, the AAMC established another task force to clarify precisely which attributes medical students should possess at the time of graduation and to set forth explicit learning objectives by which formal curricula could attain this goal. This commission, titled the Medical School Objectives Project (MSOP), published its initial report in 1998, with subsequent reports addressing special topics on contemporary issues such as communication, genetics education, and oral health education.

The first report of the MSOP defined four broad attributes that graduating physicians should have. First and foremost, "physicians must be altruistic." This heading included recommendations for formal instruction in ethics, the development of compassion and honesty, a commitment to advocacy, and an understanding of a physician's limitations, including conflicts of interest. It is revealing that this moral directive was given priority over the remaining three traditional attributes: being knowledgeable, skillful, and dutiful (AAMC 1998).

These recommendations reflected years of heated discussion, and the method and value of formal education in professionalism continue to be debated to this day. Nonetheless, they precipitated innovative courses focusing on the doctor-patient relationship and ethical principles, particularly in the preclinical years. Subsumed under names such as "The Practice of Medicine," "Medicine and Society," or "The Doctor-Patient Relationship," these courses have become a standard part of medical school curricula, even as their content continues to evolve.

While professionalism addresses the doctor-patient relationship on an individual level, culturally competent care confronts it at the level of society. Epidemiological studies had long confirmed the contribution of socioeconomic status to disease; in the 1990s, there began an exploration of factors beyond living conditions and the ability to afford health care that were contributing to racial and ethnic disparities in outcomes. Researchers began to recognize that educational, cultural, and linguistic barriers, as well as overt discrimination, were compromising access to health care, independent of financial means. The importance of folk medicine, divergent understandings of disease, and communication issues between patients and providers attained a new prominence in discussions of policy. Today, health care providers appreciate how these sociocultural differences affect every level of health care delivery, from whether an individual decides to seek care, to the type of care administered, to an individual's adherence to the care regimen (Byrd 1990; Lavizzo-Mourey and MacKenzie 1996).

Thus began a movement to address these sources of disparity by emphasizing cultural competence on systemic as well as clinical levels. Systemic innovations included an increased emphasis on interpreter services, provision of culturally appropriate health education materials, and the recruitment of a more diverse leadership and workforce. Clinical innovations emphasized educational programs for medical students, residents, and health care providers. Advocates began decrying the lack of cultural competence education in the pages of academic journals (Lum and Korenman 1994). The 1999 MSOP report, *Communication in Medicine* (AAMC 1999) included selections from a report by the Task Force on Spirituality, Cultural Issues, and End of Life Care. (This document is discussed more fully later in the context of the spirituality in medicine movement.)

Early educational programs in cultural competence were simple and straightforward. They used an approach that attempted to directly inform practitioners about the medically relevant attitudes and behaviors of various ethnic groups. For example, so that they could provide culturally competent care to Chinese patients, providers would be taught about the typical Chinese diet and family dynamics, Buddhist values, and Chinese folk remedies. While a step in the right direction, these programs were criticized for encouraging stereotypic views of ethnic groups which were unrealistic given the vast diversity of cultural groups in the U.S. population. As a result, subsequent programs employed a cross-cultural emphasis on openness and communication, with patients viewed as the ultimate authorities on their own cultural backgrounds. The provider was not expected to be omniscient about foreign cultures, but rather, sensitive to them and open to learning about them (Betancourt et al. 2003; Teal and Street 2009).

The parallel movements of medical education toward greater cultural competence and professionalism overlap. Both are essentially concerned with the articulation of the physician's self in relation to that of the patient, even as they use different means of approaching that relationship. Professionalism is the ethical and psychological counterpart of cultural competence's sociological and anthropological approach.

As professionalism and culturally competent care become part of the medical education mainstream, newer movements continue to push the envelope, at times bridging the distinctions between the personal and population-based approaches. Examples include narrative medicine, mindfulness, and integrative medicine. The borders between these movements can be nebulous, especially as many of the same advocates espouse them. Furthermore, while they may not articulate their missions in terms of spirituality per se, they emphasize self-reflection, existential experience, and openness to nontraditional forms of healing. Thus, they are clearly related to spirituality.

Briefly, narrative medicine emphasizes the importance of listening to a patient narrating his or her own experience of illness, without interruption, both as a means for the physician to better understand and address the patient's concerns and also for patients to feel that the physician appreciates their suffering. Approaching illness through narrative addresses the existential aspects of suffering while simultaneously challenging the physician's axiomatic assumptions, in order to generate a more individual and holistic approach to diagnosis and care. Furthermore, the act of narration is itself therapeutic, and the physician's participation in the patient's construction of meaning improves their therapeutic alliance. By allowing the patient to initially take charge of the therapeutic encounter, narrative medicine also encourages physicians to reflect on their own relationship to the troubling tensions inherent in medical practice (Charon 2004; Charon and Wyer 2008; Greenhalgh and Hurwitz 1999).

Mindfulness similarly finds a place in the growing recognition of the importance of physicians being self-reflective in the clinical encounter. Its advocates see the movement as a necessary step in restoring humanism. Physician self-awareness could be nurtured by various means, including individual journaling and meditations, as well as small-group discussion sessions in medical school and residency curricula (Epstein 1999; Novack, Epstein, and Paulsen 1999).

The integrative medicine movement originated in the 1990s, when medical schools began teaching complementary and alternative medicine (CAM), which has continued to grow in popularity. Its advocates emphasize that these programs should not merely acquaint physicians with popular practices, but should rather teach them the qualities that enabled CAM to inform a new paradigm within medicine. One of the earliest programs, founded at the University of Arizona in 1996, defined integrative medicine as follows: "Healing-oriented medicine that reemphasizes the relationship between patient and physician, and integrates the best of complementary and alternative medicine with the best of conventional medicine. . . . This synthesis of humanistic medicine, patient- and relationship-centered care, preventive health, allopathy, and CAM is the model for creating an improved system of health care" (Maizes et al. 2002, p. 852).

Of necessity, programs in integrative medicine tend to be comprehensive, combining aspects of professionalism and cultural competence with instruction in CAM systems, as well as experiential learning and self-reflection. In 2004, the Consortium of Academic Health Centers for Integrative Medicine published a set of core competencies for a medical school curriculum. Its members have also developed a number of courses, workshops, and readings that can be incorporated as medical school electives (Kligler et al. 2004).

The Spirituality in Medicine Movement

The movement toward spirituality in medicine began in the 1970s with the evolution of professionalism and cultural competence, as discussed above. Explicit articles on the subject began to appear in medical journals in the 1980s, and it began to be taught a few years later in elective courses and workshops at medical schools.

One of the earliest of these courses was founded by Dr. Christina Puchalski, at the George Washington School of Medicine, in 1992. In 1996 it became part of the medical school's required curriculum (Puchalski 2006). Puchalski's efforts have extended beyond her home institution. She has become one of the leading players in spirituality in medical education reform.

An important part of Puchalski's efforts has been defining the educational aims and core competencies of the spirituality in medicine movement. Puchalski served as chair of the task force that issued a report included with the third report of the MSOP in 1999, on the subject of communication, entitled "Spirituality, Cultural Issues, and End of Life Care." The report included the following learning objectives for medical students:

- The ability to elicit a spiritual history . . .
- An understanding that the spiritual dimension of people's lives is an avenue for compassionate care giving
- The ability to apply the understanding of a patient's spirituality and cultural beliefs and behaviors to appropriate clinical contexts (e.g., in prevention, case formulation, treatment planning, challenging clinical situations)
- Knowledge of the research data on the impact of spirituality on health and on health care outcomes . . .
- An understanding of, and respect for, the role of clergy and other spiritual leaders, and culturally based healers and care providers, and how to communicate and/or collaborate with them on behalf of patients' physical and/or spiritual needs
- An understanding of their own spirituality and how it can be nurtured as part of their professional growth, promotion of their wellbeing, and the basis of their calling as a physician. (AAMC 1999, p. 26)

These objectives explicate that while the movement is deeply concerned with meeting the spiritual needs of patients (akin to cultural competence), it also aims to address the role of spirituality in physicians' lives. In 2001, Puchalski helped found the George Washington Institute for Spirituality and Health (GWish), which sponsored a conference on "national competencies in spirituality and health education initiative" in 2009 to refine these objectives and formulate outcome measures for spirituality education programs (GWish 2009d).

How to attain these learning objectives has been the project of Puchalski and other educators over the past two decades. In the process, they have encountered resistance. Academic medicine is, to a significant degree, still dominated by attitudes implicit in the biomedical model that value scientific knowledge over so-called soft subjects such as social sciences, ethics, and communication skills. These attitudes are reinforced by licensing examinations that demand factual knowledge, easily tested in the multiple-choice format. Curriculum directors are often rightfully concerned that soft subjects occupy valuable time and space needed to cover an ever-growing body of biomedical knowledge. Because spirituality is defined so broadly, they assume that it is already addressed in courses on professionalism or cultural competence.

There is additional resistance to spirituality in particular. Prominent scientific critics such as Richard Dawkins have painted religion as an inherently biased phenomenon defined by irrationality, and anything associated with it as the antithesis of scientific progress. No doubt influenced by such rhetoric, many physicians and administrators feel that spirituality has no place in a medical curriculum or in medical practice. Despite a significant body of research arguing to the contrary (Anandarajah and Hight 2001; Mueller, Plevak, and Rummans 2001), they do not see religion and spirituality as directly contributing to human health and therefore consider it irrelevant. This is probably related to the fact that physicians are less likely to consider themselves religious or spiritual compared with the general population (Curlin et al. 1994).

However, the resistance is not simply a matter of discomfort; it is often articulated in ethical terms as a concern about the place of spirituality in medicine and medical education. There is a palpable discomfort with even bringing up the subject with patients, as many physicians assume that doing so might lead to a request for spiritual guidance. Responding to such a request outside their area of expertise can be seen as an abuse of their status as medical professionals. The possibility of addressing an important patient concern is thus countered by the possibility of doing harm by confronting issues about which physicians are ignorant (Scheurich 2003; Sloan, Bagiella, and Powell 1999).

Furthermore, any discussion of religion or spirituality may be regarded as akin to proselytizing. Studies have demonstrated that physicians who identify themselves as religious or spiritual are more likely to support discussing such subjects with their patients compared with those who identify themselves as minimally religious or spiritual (Curlin et al. 2006). Institutions providing major financial support for GWish, such as the John Templeton Foundation and the F.I.S.H. Foundation, have both generated controversy—the Templeton Foundation for the strong religious convictions of its founder, and the F.I.S.H. Foundation for its articulated mission "to touch others' lives with the love of Christ" (F.I.S.H. Foundation 2011).

Teaching medical students about religion might similarly be considered proselytizing. Critics observe that lecturers tend to be religious themselves and may be espousing their own religious values. Furthermore, students already socialized into a biomedical culture and sensitized to the issue of professional boundaries often resist courses in religion and spirituality.

In response to this resistance, educational programs make a concerted effort to address themselves to scenarios that are clearly relevant for clinicians. What should you do if your patient asks you why God is punishing her? What should you do if a patient refuses medical care because of his religious or spiritual beliefs? While the conclusions of spirituality-in-medicine advocates may not always appeal to cynics, it becomes difficult to object to discussions of spirituality when patients themselves initiate them (Curlin et al. 2006). Another response is to cite patient surveys indicating that many patients want their physicians to ask about their religious or spiritual beliefs (Daaleman and Nease 1994). Finally, advocates emphasize the importance of open-ended questions and tentative exploration rather than emphatic recommendations in the context of a clinical encounter (Lo et al. 2002).

Two Approaches: Integrated and Separate Courses

Two main approaches have developed to incorporate spiritual medicine into medical school curricula. One is to integrate it into preexisting courses on professionalism, cultural competence, and related subjects. The other is to offer separate courses on spirituality in medicine.

Many curricular reforms supported by GWish have incorporated spirituality in a variety of formats, including readings, small-group discussions, journaling, and history taking (GWish 2009a). This approach has both logistical and philosophical advantages. By drawing on the resources of other courses, it avoids much of the hassle involved in organizing a separate course, such as recruiting faculty and carving out space in the curriculum. Furthermore, rather than segregating the topic, it serves to demonstrate its relevance to various aspects of medical practice. However, the lack of advocates for spirituality education within academic medicine renders this strategy difficult to implement. The course directors who make the ultimate decisions about what material is to be covered often do not consider spirituality a priority. Similarly, individuals teaching courses may not feel comfortable with addressing spiritual issues and therefore may skim over relevant topics when they appear.

One simple way to integrate spirituality into the curriculum is to teach taking the patient's spiritual history as part of existing courses on history taking. Just as there are standard questions for addressing difficult issues such as drug use or sexual practices, several schema exist for the spiritual history. The HOPE questions ask specifically about a patient's sources of *h*ope, affiliation with *o*rganized religion, feelings of *p*ersonal spirituality, and the *e*ffects of the above on their approach to medical care (Anandarajah and Hight 2001). The SPIRIT scheme addresses a patient's *s*piritual belief *s*ystem, *p*ersonal spirituality, *i*ntegration with a spiritual community, *r*itualized practices and *r*estrictions, *i*mplications of the above for their medical care, and *t*erminal events planning (Maugans 1996). GWish similarly developed a FICA acronym that can be applied to a spiritual history as well as personal reflection (GWish 2009c). Studies have demonstrated that teaching such questions to medical students helps them appreciate the relevance of spiritual history taking and spirituality to clinical practice (King et al. 2004).

At Harvard Medical School, several courses integrate spirituality to some degree. These courses originated in the reforms of former dean Daniel Tosteson, who in 1985 introduced a radically reformed preclinical curriculum known as the "New Pathway." The New Pathway was designed to minimize lectures in favor of small-group, problem-based learning that integrated clinical concepts into the first two years of medical school. It also introduced a series of "Patient-Doctor" courses to teach history taking and physical examination skills. In 1987, the New Pathway was extended to the entire class, dividing the student body into four academic societies to facilitate interactions among students of different classes and medical faculty. A fifth society, affiliated with the Massachusetts institute of Technology, followed a separate curriculum focusing on health and science technology (HST). The New Pathway was reformed in 2006 to introduce mandatory courses in subjects such as ethics and social medicine and to have students begin their clinical clerkships two months earlier, in May of their second year (Tosteson 1990).

The New Pathway and HST programs both begin with a two-week course called "Introduction to the Profession," which includes journal exercises and small-group sessions encouraging students to consider the changes that are about to occur in their lives. Another opportunity for reflection is a donor memorial service held at the end of the first-year anatomy course. The reflective format returns in the third year with Patient-Doctor III, a bimonthly series of seminars in which students reflect on difficult scenarios encountered in clinical practice, such as dysfunctional team dynamics, end-of-life issues, uncertainty, and more recently, mindfulness. Finally, while the seminar-based course on ethics encourages a more philosophical approach to moral quandaries, it includes discussions about topics that traditionally invoke religious or spiritual arguments, such as physician-assisted suicide, reproductive rights, and genetic testing.

The New Pathway includes other courses in which spirituality might be addressed even if course directors have not done so historically. Psychosocial issues are already integrated into many of the cases in the core science courses, but more in terms of ethnicity or socioeconomic circumstances. Religion and spirituality tend not to be addressed directly, a trend echoed in the mandatory social medicine course. Finally, Patient-Doctor I, which teaches history taking, includes a session on patient support systems, including religious and spiritual beliefs, although it does not emphasize spiritual history taking.

The second approach to teaching spirituality in medicine, which tends to be more popular in practice, is by means of separate courses and workshops. The advantage of this approach is that it allows faculty more complete control over the material and facilitates creative teaching methods that might not be suited to a traditional classroom setting. However, it has the distinct disadvantage of typically resulting in elective rather than required courses. As medical curricula become increasingly crowded, it becomes progressively difficult to attract students to such elective courses, and students who do not have an appreciation for the relevance of spirituality in medicine will not apply in any case. Furthermore, this segregation arguably reinforces the idea that spirituality in medicine is a special interest rather than a core competency.

The possibilities for how to develop such courses are myriad, and one major obstacle encountered by course directors is how to limit themselves. Spirituality in medicine is defined broadly, and attempting to distill the field into a course of a few hours' or weeks' duration is an exercise in futility. Courses also use a variety of teaching modalities, including lectures, panels, small-group discussions, journaling, incorporation of art or music, meditation, and fieldwork components. It is therefore impossible to summarize a general approach to such courses, especially because there is scant literature that goes into the details of the courses offered (Fortin and Barnett 2004). Therefore, I focus here on several elective courses that currently exist at Harvard Medical School.

Harvard's only current course with the word *spirituality* in its title is an elective offered by the editors of this volume, John Peteet and Michael D'Ambra, on which this collection is based. The course has its origins in a 1999 course by Herbert Benson, director emeritus of the Benson-Henry Institute for Mind Body Medicine at Massachusetts General Hospital. While the course was initially popular, drawing almost 50 students its first year, some felt that it lacked conceptual coherence or clinical relevance, addressing topics as disparate as Native American Spirituality and attachment theory. It was suspended after several years. The course was resurrected in 2004 by Peteet, who had served as a tutor in the original course, and D'Ambra. After a student in the first year objected that the course was biased toward individuals with personal faith, a third course director, Ed Lowenstein, an atheist, was invited to join (J. R. Peteet, personal communication).

The course was originally directed primarily at medical students. However, the 2006 reforms of the New Pathway significantly reduced the time students have available for electives, resulting in many courses having difficulty attracting sufficient enrollment. The course directors responded to this by opening enrollment to house staff, faculty, chaplains, and divinity school students, an innovation that has resulted in rich discussions. The course alternates between lectures and small-group discussions based on readings on topics reflected by the chapters in this collection. Participants discuss their readings with the class; those taking the course for credit must present a final paper based on a fieldwork experience to the group at the final session. Suggestions for fieldwork include shadowing a chaplain, interviewing a patient or practitioner about how spirituality influences their approach to care, or exploring spirituality-based healing modalities such as Alcoholics Anonymous.

The course directors have found that several considerations seem to facilitate a rewarding experience for participants. The first is to attempt a balance between theory and experience, the general and the particular, and the needs of the patient and those of the clinician. While readings tend to be more academic in nature and speakers more personal, the diversity of the speakers (primarily practitioners representing different worldviews and/or religious traditions) helps balance these competing claims. The second is to maintain, as much as possible, a consistent group of student participants, preferably representing diverse types of religiosity or spirituality. This not only leads to complex discussions of recurring topics and themes but also fosters a sense of community and trust that allows for open and honest exchange on potentially volatile issues. Finally, time for discussion after lectures is vital, especially as speakers are deliberately presenting their own particular and potentially biased viewpoints. Providing time for participants to express disagreement or frustration is also important to maintaining supportive group dynamics.

Several other electives address spirituality in different ways. "The Healer's Art" is a reflection-based course developed by Rachel Remen, a major advocate of integrative medicine, in which students meet in groups of four to discuss their personal experiences as they relate to themes of self-care, grief, wonder, and meaning. In "Living with Life-Threatening Illness," students follow a single patient for several months while participating in structured learning experiences on topics such as responses to suffering, grief and loss, spiritual concerns, and ethical dilemmas. "Mind-Body Medicine" explores several CAM modalities while also requiring that students participate in yoga, meditation, or a related experience during the course. All of these courses have experienced declining enrollment since 2006.

The courses mentioned above tend to be directed toward students in the first two years of medical school. Yet the recent example of Harvard's "Spirituality in Medicine" course demonstrates that courses may benefit from participation by learners at a variety of levels. These courses also provide opportunity for incorporating spirituality into graduate and continuing education. House staff and faculty might benefit both as participants and as preceptors for courses aimed at medical students. Furthermore, residency programs—particularly those in psychiatry (Lawrence and Duggal 2001; McCarthy and Peteet 2003), primary care (King and Crisp 2005), oncology (Boston, Puchalski, and O'Donnell 2006), and palliative care (Marr, Billings, and Weissman 2007)—are increasingly incorporating their own courses in spirituality. Some of these are supported by GWish grants (GWish 2009b). Extending spirituality training into the residency years not only helps reinforce the core competencies that have a tendency to wane in the midst of heavy patient loads, but also allows programs to address specific issues that tend to be particular to a given specialty.

The spirituality in medicine movement has grown and developed considerably over the past decade, thanks to the tireless efforts of its advocates. It is far from established, however, and continuous work is likely to be necessary to maintain this development and prevent it from sharing the fate of the "comprehensive medicine" reforms of the 1940s–1950s. In addition to continuing to develop and implement curricular reforms, advocates will probably need to continue research demonstrating the relevancy of religion and spirituality to health and healing to bolster their arguments as they continue to fight for space in the curriculum. They will also need to address the difficulty of communication among educators involved in curriculum development. While informal communication occurs within a given institution, no journal is currently dedicated to spirituality in medicine, and few articles are specifically devoted to the teaching of spirituality in medicine. GWish is currently working to develop such a publication, as well as a Spirituality and Health Online Education and Resource Center (SOERCE) to provide educators with access to peer-reviewed discussion of curricula designs (GWish 2009e). Another resource that has hitherto been underused is the rich discussion of this topic within other fields, including chaplaincy, nursing, and social work. A collaborative effort with experts from these fields, for education as well as for the implementation of spirituality in clinical care, could be promising.

REFERENCES

AAMC (Association of American Medical Colleges). 1932. *Final Report of the Commission on Medical Education.* New York: *Office of the Director of the Study.*

———. 1984. *Physicians for the Twenty-First Century: The GPEP Report;* Report *of the Panel on the General Professional Education of the Physician and College Preparation for Medicine.* Washington, DC.

———. 1998. *Learning Objectives for Medical Student Education: Guidelines for Medical Schools.* Medical School Objectives Project, Report I. Washington, DC. https://services.aamc.org/publications/index.cfm?fuseaction=Product.displayForm&prd_id=198&prv_id=239. Accessed 28 Nov. 2009.

———. 1999. *Contemporary Issues in Medicine: Communication in Medicine.* Medical School Objectives Project, Report III. Washington, DC. https://services.aamc.org/publications/index.cfm?fuseaction=Product.displayForm&prd_id=200&prv_id=241. Accessed 28 Nov. 2009.

Anandarajah, G., and E. Hight. 2001. Spirituality and medical practice: Using the HOPE questions as a practical tool for spiritual assessment. *American Family Physician* 3:81–89.

Betancourt, J. R., A. R. Green, J. E. Carrillo, and A. F. Owusu. 2003. Defining cultural competence: A practical framework for addressing racial/ethnic disparities in health and health care. *Public Health Reports* 118:293–302.

Boston, P., C. M. Puchalski, and J. F. O'Donnell. 2006. American Association for Cancer Education membership perspectives of spirituality in cancer education. *Journal of Cancer Education* 21:8–12.

Byrd, W. M. 1990. Race, biology, and healthcare: Reassessing a relationship. *Journal of Health Care for the Poor and Underserved* 1:278–96.

Charon, R. 2004. Narrative and medicine. *New England Journal of Medicine* 350:862–64.

Charon, R., and P. Wyer. 2008. Narrative evidence based medicine. *Lancet* 371:296–97.

Curlin, F. A., M. H. Chin, S. A. Sellergren, C. J. Roach, and J. D. Lantos. 2006. The association of physicians' religious characteristics with their attitudes and self-reported behaviors regarding religion and spirituality in the clinical encounter. *Medical Care* 44:446–53.

Curlin, F. A., J. D. Lantos, C. J. Roach, S. A. Sellergren, and M. H. Chin. 1994. Religious characteristics of U.S. physicians: A national survey. *Journal of General Internal Medicine* 20:629–34.

Daaleman, T. P., and D. E. Nease. 1994. Patient attitudes regarding physician inquiry into spiritual and religious issues. *Journal of Family Practice* 39:564–68.

Engel, G. L. 1977. The need for a new medical model: A challenge for biomedicine. *Science* 196:129–36.

Epstein, R. 1999. Mindful practice. *JAMA* 282:833–39.

Feudtner, C., D. A. Christakis, and N. A. Christakis. 1994. Do clinical clerks suffer ethical erosion? Students' perceptions of their ethical environment and personal development. *Academic Medicine* 69:670–79.

F.I.S.H. Foundation. 2011. Our Mission. www.fishfoundationinc.org/mission.html. Accessed Feb. 2011.

Flexner, A. 1910. *Medical Education in the United States and Canada*. New York: Carnegie Foundation for the Advancement of Teaching.

Fortin, A. H., and K. G. Barnett. 2004. Medical school curricula in spirituality and medicine. *JAMA* 291:2883.

Greenhalgh, T., and B. Hurwitz. 1999. Narrative based medicine: Why study narrative? *BMJ* 318:48–50.

GWish (George Washington Institute for Spirituality and Health). 2009a. Award for Curriculum Development in Medical Schools. www.gwumc.edu/gwish/awards/medschawardees.cfm. Accessed Aug. 2009.

———. 2009b. Curricular and Residency Training Program Awards. www.gwumc.edu/gwish/awards/index.cfm. Accessed Aug. 2009.

———. 2009c. FICA Spiritual History Tool. www.gwumc.edu/gwish/clinical/fica.cfm. Accessed Aug. 2009.

———. 2009d. National Competencies. www.gwumc.edu/gwish/education/national competencies.cfm. Accessed Aug. 2009.

———. 2009e. SOERCE. www.gwumc.edu/gwish/soerce/index.cfm. Accessed Aug. 2009.

Hafferty, F. W., and R. Franks. 1994. The hidden curriculum, ethics teaching, and the structure of medical education. *Academic Medicine* 69:861–71.

Kendall, P. L., and G. G. Reader. 1988. Innovations in medical education of the 1950s contrasted with those of the 1970s and 1980s. *Journal of Health and Social Behavior* 29:279–93.

King, D. E., A. Blue, R. Mallin, and C. Thiedke. 2004. Implementation and assessment of a spiritual-history-taking curriculum in the first year of medical school. *Teaching and Learning in Medicine* 16:64–68.

King, D. E., and J. Crisp. 2005. Spirituality and health care education in family medicine residency programs. *Family Medicine* 37:399–403.

Kleinman, A., L. Eisenberg, and B. Good. 1978. Culture, illness, and care: Clinical lessons from anthropological and cross-cultural research. *Annals of Internal Medicine* 88:251–58.

Kligler, B., V. Maizes, S. Schachter, C. M. Park, T. Gaudet, R. Benn, R. Lee, and R. N. Remen.

2004. Core competencies in integrative medicine for medical school curricula: A proposal. *Academic Medicine* 79:521–31.

Lavizzo-Mourey, R. J., and E. MacKenzie. 1996. Cultural competence: An essential hybrid for delivering high quality care in the 1990's and beyond. *Transactions of the American Clinical and Climatological Association* 107:226–37.

Lawrence, R. M., and A. Duggal. 2001. Spirituality in psychiatric education and training. *Journal of the Royal Society of Medicine* 94:303–5.

Lo, B., D. Ruston, L. W. Kates, R. M. Arnold, C. B. Cohen, K. Faber-Langendoen, S. Z. Pantilat, et al. 2002. Discussing religious and spiritual issues at the end of life: A practical guide for physicians. *JAMA* 287:749–54.

Ludmerer, K. 1999. *Time to Heal: American Medical Education from the Turn of the Century to the Era of Managed Care*. New York: Oxford University Press.

Lum, C. K., and S. G. Korenman. 1994. Cultural-sensitivity training in US medical schools. *Academic Medicine* 69:239–40.

Maizes, V., C. Schneider, I. Bell, and A. Weil. 2002. Integrative medical education: Development and implementation of a comprehensive curriculum at the University of Arizona. *Academic Medicine* 77:851–60.

Marr, L., J. A. Billings, and D. E. Weissman. 2007. Spirituality training for palliative care fellows. *Journal of Palliative Medicine* 10:169–77.

Maugans, T. A. 1996. The SPIRITual history. *Archives of Family Medicine* 5:11–16.

McCarthy, M. K., and J. R. Peteet. 2003. Teaching residents about religion and spirituality. *Harvard Review of Psychiatry* 11:225–28.

McQuade, J. S. 1991. The medical malpractice crisis: Reflections on the alleged causes and proposed cures. Discussion paper. *Journal of the Royal Society of Medicine* 84:408–11.

Mueller, P. S., D. J. Plevak, and T. A. Rummans. 2001. Religious involvement, spirituality, and medicine: Implications for clinical practice. *Mayo Clinic Proceedings* 76:1225–35.

Neville, A. J., and G. R. Norman. 2007. PBL in the undergraduate MD program at McMaster University: Three iterations in three decades. *Academic Medicine* 82:370–74.

Newsweek. 1987. Malpractice suits: Doctors under siege. Special Report. *Newsweek*, 26 Jan. 1987, p. 62.

New York Times. 1987. The legacy of Libby Zion (editorial). *New York Times*. 8 June.

Novack, D. H., R. M. Epstein, and R. H. Paulsen. 1999. Toward creating physician-healers: Fostering medical students' self-awareness, personal growth, and well-being. *Academic Medicine* 74:516–20.

Peabody, F. W. 1927. The care of the patient. *JAMA* 88:877–82.

Philibert, I., P. Friedmann, and W. T. Williams. 2002. New requirements for resident duty hours. *JAMA* 288:1112–14.

Puchalski, C. M. 2006. Spirituality and medicine: Curricula in medical education. *Journal of Cancer Education* 21:14–18.

Scheurich, N. 2003. Reconsidering spirituality and medicine. *Academic Medicine* 78:356–60.

Silver, H. K., and A. D. Glicksen. 1990. Medical student abuse: Incidence, severity, and significance. *JAMA* 263:527–32.

Sloan, R. P., E. Bagiella, and T. Powell. 1999. Religion, spirituality, and medicine. *Lancet* 353:664–67.

Teal, C. R., and R. L. Street. 2009. Critical elements of culturally competent communication in the medical encounter: A review and model. *Social Science and Medicine* 68:533–43.

Tosteson, D. C. 1990. New pathways in general medical education. *New England Journal of Medicine* 322:234–38.

Welch, M. 1998. Required curricula in diversity and cross-cultural medicine: The time is now. *JAMWA* 53:121–24.

Index

Page numbers in italics refer to figures and tables.